Studies in Disorders of Communication

General Editors:

David Crysal
Honorary Professor of Linguistics, University College of North Wales, Bangor

Ruth Lesser
Head of Speech Department, University of Newcastle-upon-tyne

Margaret Snowing
Principal, National Hospitals College of Speech Sciences, London

Studies in Disorders of Communication

General Editors

Pragmatic Disability in Children

MICHAEL F. McTEAR
AND GINA CONTI-RAMSDEN

STUDIES IN DISORDERS OF COMMUNICATION

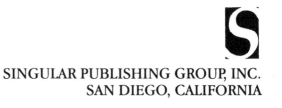

SINGULAR PUBLISHING GROUP, INC.
SAN DIEGO, CALIFORNIA

©Whurr Publishers Ltd 1992
19b Compton Terrace
London N1 2UN
England

Published and Distributed in the
United States and Canada by
SINGULAR PUBLISHING GROUP, INC.
4284 41st Street
San Diego, California 92105

Library of Congress Cataloging in Publication Data
McTear. Michael.
    Pragmatic disability in children / Michael F. McTear and Gina
Conti-Ramsden.
        p. cm.
    Includes bibliographical references and index.
    ISBN 1-879105-56-X
    1. Language disorders in children. 2. Pragmatics. I. Conti-
Ramsden. Gina. II. Title.
RJ496. L35M39 1991   91-31030
618. 92'855--dc20   CIP

Photoset by Stephen Cary
Printed and bound in the UK by Athenaeum Ltd, Newcastle upon
Tyne

Preface

In the last decade the term "pragmatics" has probably become the most widely used word among those interested in language development and language disabilities. There has been a variety of efforts to refine it, study it, observe its development in children, and, in addition, examine what happens when young people have difficulties with the pragmatic aspects of language.

One of our aims in this book is to discuss the impact of pragmatics in the study of what we term "pragmatic disabilities", in an effort to integrate our knowledge and research on normal language development with that of a typical language learner. A second aim of the book is to provide a broader framework within which "pragmatic disabilities" are studied. A linguistic framework is examined but also alternative explanations such as sociocognitive factors and emotional effects are considered. Finally, a third aim of the book is to demystify some of the information related to pragmatics and pragmatic disabilities. We have attempted to provide a thorough review of the field in a clear, simple, and well-exemplified fashion in order to reach researchers, practitioners, and students alike.

In writing this book we have drawn from the work of many scholars. Our debt to them is acknowledged in the references but we would like to mention especially Dorothy Bishop, Catherine Snow and the late Carol Prutting for their pioneer work on pragmatic development and disabilities. We would also like to thank David Crystal and Dorothy Bishop who read earlier versions of the book and provided us with many helpful comments and ideas.

Needless to say, this work would not have been possible without the support and encouragement of our respective families, who showed patience and understanding during the many hours dedicated to the book.

Dedications

Gina: To John, Michael, Frances, and my mother Alicia; for their smiles at the end of each day.
Michael: To Sandra, Siobhan, Paul, Anna, and Rachel; for their love and sense of fun.

General Preface

This series focuses upon disorders of speech language and communication, bringing together the techniques of analysis, assessment and treatment which are pertinent to the area. It aims to cover cognitive, linguistic, social and education aspects of language disability, and therefore has relevance within a number of disciplines. These include speech therapy, the education of children and adults with special needs, teachers of the deaf, teachers of English as a second language and of foreign languages, and educational and clinical psychology. The research and clinical findings from these various areas can usefully inform one another and, therefore, we hope one of the main functions of this series will be to put people within one profession in touch with developments in another. Thus, it is our editorial policy to ask authors to consider the implications of their findings for professions outside their own and for fields with which they have not been primarily concerned. We hope to engender an integrated approach to theory and practice and to produce a much-needed emphasis on the description and analysis of language as such, as well as on the provision of specific techniques of therapy, remediation and rehabilitation

Whilst it has been our aim to restrict the series to the study of language disability, its scope goes considerably beyond this. Many previously neglected topics have been included where these seem to benefit from contemporary research in linguistics, psychology, medicine, sociology, education and English studies. Each volume puts its subject matter in perspective and provides an introductory slant to its presentation. In this way we hope to provide specialized studies which can be used as texts for components of teaching courses at undergraduate and postgraduate levels, as well as material directly applicable to the needs of professional workers.

David Crystal
Ruth Lesser
Margaret Snowling

Contents

Contents

Chapter 1
Introducing
Pragmatic Disability

Pragmatics has become one of the keywords of the past decade for speech–language pathologists. It is only necessary to scan the contents' pages of journals or take notice of the themes of conferences, courses and workshops to become aware of this new perspective on language and communication. Thus increasingly we come across studies of children's discourse skills, pragmatic abilities, functional uses of language, and communicative competence. Equally there is a growing number of studies concerned with problems and difficulties experienced by some children in these aspects of language use. One consequence of this development is a heightened awareness of the complexities of everyday communication. Pragmatic issues are being increasingly addressed in clinical practice, in terms of changing perspectives on how certain types of language disorder are viewed as well as in terms of new ideas for assessment and intervention.

However, despite all this interest and activity there is a tremendous lack of clarity about pragmatics – what the term means, how it is relevant to speech–language pathologists, what sort of disability might be described as pragmatic. Around 1985 there was a lively debate in the British College of Speech Therapists' Bulletin about pragmatics – in particular, about the meaning of the term "semantic–pragmatic disorder". Some of this discussion highlighted the amount of confusion that exists in the current understanding of many aspects of language use and in the range of difficulties experienced by some language-disabled children. This debate is still active, although the focus has sharpened somewhat as some of the issues have become clearer. At the same time, much remains to be resolved. Within linguistic theory there is controversy over whether some of the aspects of language use studied in pragmatics fall within the scope of linguistics or whether they belong more generally to disciplines such as communication studies. For those concerned with children who have difficulties with various aspects of the use of language, there is the question of whether the difficulties are primarily linguistic, cognitive, social, or emotional–affective. There is even the question of whether there is such a thing as "pragmatic disorder" or whether some of the observed problems in the use of language are manifestations of other well-documented disorders, such as autism.

The term "pragmatic" is often used to encompass those aspects of language use that are subject to systematic variation according to the social context. Children with problems in recognizing and satisfying the social rules of language are usually described as having *pragmatic disabilities*. These children often have difficulty in school, with making friends and coping with everyday social interaction. Nonetheless, their problems are not always obvious and there is an urgent need for more research in this area.

Pragmatic issues are being increasingly addressed in clinical practice, in terms of changing perspectives on how certain types of language disorder are viewed as well as in terms of new ideas for assessment and intervention.

It is the purpose of this book to address these issues and to provide some insight and direction for those practitioners and researchers who are professionally concerned with those children having difficulties in using language for everyday communication. The range of problems that might be included under the term "pragmatic disability" is examined and a review provided of research that is relevant to the understanding of these issues. This review will serve as a foundation for the remainder of the book, in which the development of pragmatic abilities in children with normal as well as with atypical language abilities is examined; studies of parent–child and clinician–child interactions are described; and methods reviewed for the assessment of pragmatic disability, implications for treatment, and prospects for further research.

Before proceeding, however, it will be helpful to examine some examples of conversations involving pragmatically disabled children in order to illustrate more clearly the sorts of problems that are involved.

Some examples

Many examples have been reported of children whose use of language tends to disrupt normal conversation in complex ways. They may fail to respond appropriately to what their dialogue partner has just said; they may pay undue attention to the literal meaning of what is said rather than its intended meaning; they may be unaware of what their listener knows and does not know; they engage in odd associations and reasoning; they are unable to detect and repair misunderstandings. These and other aspects of pragmatic disability are looked at in greater detail in Chapters 4, 5 and 6. For the present, some typical examples are presented and briefly analysed.

Example 1

The speech–language pathologist and an 8-year-old boy are sitting talking:

T: What's wrong with Miss X (child's teacher)?
        Why isn't she here?
C: She's in bed.
T: She's sick?
C: Yes, she's in bed.
T: Oh dear!
        How do you think she's feeling if she's in bed?
C: Ehm ... ehm ...
        Alright.
T: You think she's feeling alright?
C: No ... ehm ... maybe.
T: Maybe she's feeling alright.
        But if she's in bed and she is a bit sick, how do you think she feels
        – sad or happy?
C: Sad.
T: I would say so, I would say sad.
        A bit sad and a bit tired.
        Maybe we can send her a card.
C: Send her a card?

We can note that this child is able to take turns and responds to the clinician's questions. However, there is something inappropriate about the content of the child's turns. For example, he says his teacher is alright when she is sick in bed.

It could be argued that this is a simple misunderstanding or confusion and, of course, more examples would be necessary before anything more definite could be concluded about this child's level of understanding. Some potentially useful evidence could be the degree of hesitation at crucial points in the conversation. For example, this child hesitates when he seems to be unsure of the implications of being in bed and being sick. Similarly, when he is not sure what to say after the therapist asks "You think she's feeling alright", he hesitates and mumbles "No ... ehm ... maybe". A number of similar examples would indicate that the child may have problems in understanding. Further investigation could show that the child has problems in relating one piece of information to another in order to make sense of what is going on. For example, it seems that this child does not see the connection between being sick and feeling sad. Yet further analysis might show that the child is unable to put himself in the other person's perspective and understand that other people have beliefs and feelings that are different from his own. Another issue is that the child may be unaware of socially relevant norms and customs. For example, in response to the clinician's "Maybe we can send her a card", he says "Send her a card?", which could indicate that he does not understand why they should wish to send his teacher a card.

Of course, none of these interpretations can stand on their own. Further evidence and careful analysis is necessary. However, from this short example we can see how it is possible to discover aspects of a child's pragmatic problems from examination of conversations involving the child. In later chapters there will be extensive expansion on the sorts of problems merely hinted at here.

Example 2

The teacher and a 9 year old are looking at a picture of a baby with dirty diapers

T: Why does a baby have to wear a diaper?
        Do you know?
C: Yeah.
T: Why?
C: He can't go in the toilet.
T: He can't go in the toilet.
        So what happens to his diapers, do they get clean or dirty?
C: Clean.
T: Are they clean? (pointing to picture)
C: Yes.
T: What does the baby do in the diaper?
C: Toilet.
T: That's right.
        The baby's toilet is pretty much the diaper, isn't it?
C: Yeah.
T: What would happen if the baby didn't have a diaper?
C: Don't know.

Again this conversation appears to be odd as the child does not seem to be responding in the expected ways. This child is aware that he needs to respond in order to keep up his end of the conversation. To the teacher's question "So what happens to the diapers, do they get dirty or clean?" he can respond either "clean" or "dirty". However, the response "clean" does not make sense in this context, which could lead to the suspicion that the child has difficulties with reasoning – in particular, with making the connection between going to the toilet in a diaper and the state of cleanliness of that diaper.

It could, of course, be argued that this and some of the other questions put to this child are simply too difficult and that the child is forced into a strategy of saying whatever comes to mind rather than working out the most appropriate answer. To be sure of this, we would need to know more information about the child, for example, whether the child had severe learning difficulties and what specifically those difficulties were. In this particular case, the child did not have any such learning difficulties, but nevertheless was frequently unable to make connections (or inferences) and to adopt the perspective of other people.

Example 3

The adult asks whether the child goes home every day after school:

C: We go home every day.
A: Do you go home every day?
C: Yes.
A: Where do you live Stephen?
C: London.
A: So you don't go home every day.

At first glance this example appears odd because of what the teacher says. The child makes a statement about going home which the teacher queries. Then the teacher asks where the child lives and, when the child replies "London", the teacher contradicts the child's previous statement about going home every day.

However, in order to appreciate what has gone wrong here, it is necessary to have some background knowledge. This conversation takes place in Nottingham, which is about 3 hours' traveling time from London, the child's home. It is unlikely that the child spends 6 hours a day travelling to and from school. For this reason the child's answer is implausible. Of course, it could be argued here that the child has simply misunderstood the word *home* to mean the place where he stays during the week. Again, further evidence would be required to establish whether the child often had problems with reasoning in similar contexts. (Note: this example is taken from an article by Stubbs (1986) which includes many more examples as well as a clear discussion of pragmatic disability.)

Example 4

The adult is talking to the child about camping:

A: Did you go camping in the woods?
C: Camping in the woods? (shouts)
A: Yeah, did you ever do that?
C: Yeah, he ever do that.

This example is taken from a case study of an 8-year-old boy with severe communication difficulties (Greenlee, 1981). In this study it was noted that 40 percent of questions to the child received no response, while 25 percent received inappropriate or unrelated responses. We can see how the child's first response to the adult's question is odd. Although the child's utterance might have been intended as a request for confirmation, (e.g. "Are you asking me about camping in the woods?"), we can note the inappropriate loudness. Further evidence that something is wrong would be if the child frequently echoed back questions rather than responding to them. Another source of evidence is the remainder of the conversation. We can see from the next exchange that things do not improve. The adult does confirm that she is asking about camping, but the child's response is odd because of the use of pronouns. This was again a frequent problem with this child, so that it was often not possible to know whether he was talking about himself or about some other person. A further exchange illustrates this problem, which is exacerbated by his failure to respond appropriately to the *when* question:

A: When are you going home?
C: Um – he IS going home

Example 5

The child is discussing with his speech–language pathologist a forthcoming sports day at school:

A: Which race would you like to be in?
C: I like to be in Longtree in the sports day.
        (Longtree is a town several miles from the school)
A: In Longtree?
C: Yes.
A: What do you mean?
C: I mean something.
A: Is there a sports day in Longtree?
C: There is not – there is a sports day in Abbeyvale.
        (Abbeyvale is the school)
A: Then what's Longtree got to do with it?
C: Nothing.
A: Then why did you mention it?
C: Indeed I did mention it.
A: Why did you mention it?
C: I don't know

This example, taken from McTear (1985a), is similar to the previous examples in that it shows that the child's responses are inappropriate and inconsistent, because it is unclear where the child intended to be on sports day. The example also shows how difficult it can be to resolve such misunderstandings: the clinician's attempts at clarification only result in further misunderstandings until the conversation develops into a complete tangle out of which neither the clinician nor the child can successfully emerge.

Examples such as these could be multiplied ad infinitum. Indeed it is common at workshops on pragmatic disability to exchange anecdotes involving similar odd uses of language by children. It might be helpful at this point, however, to indicate some of the main characteristics of children described as having pragmatic disability. The following is a typical list (Rapin and Allen, 1983; Bishop and Rosenbloom, 1987):

- Early history may include echolalia, jargon, poor symbolic skills, poor social relationships, hyperactivity.
- Delayed speech and language development, but once language develops it appears clear and fluent, with syntax and phonology developing fairly normally but with problems in semantics and pragmatics, for example:
  - odd associations and reasoning;
  - tangential or inappropriate remarks;
  - undue attention to literal rather than underlying meaning;
  - problems in understanding normal conversation, for example, descriptions of sequences of everyday events that are related temporally or causally;
  - lack of awareness of what knowledge is shared between speaker and hearer.
- Poor social skills – either withdrawn or eccentric and over-friendly.

These aspects of pragmatic disability are examined in greater detail throughout this book. But first it is important to attempt to define the term "pragmatics" and to give an overview of those issues that fall within this area.

What is pragmatics?

Unfortunately, there is no straightforward answer to this question. One approach might be along the following lines: pragmatics is an area of linguistics, so a reasonable place to start might be by examining the ways in which linguists relate pragmatics to other areas of linguistic enquiry. Thus the position might be taken that phonology is the study of the sound patterns of a language, syntax is concerned with how words can be combined into sentences, semantics is the study of meaning, and pragmatics examines how language is used.

However, if we examine textbooks on pragmatics or issues of the *Journal of Pragmatics,* we will find that the study of the use of language encompasses a wide range of phenomena, including: the structural analysis of texts; functional aspects of language usage; descriptions of speech events; accounts of how utterances are used to accomplish social actions; studies of how people process spoken and written texts; and analyses of how people engage in everyday conversation. Moreover, not all of these issues fall neatly within the concerns of linguistics and in any case many aspects of language usage are studied in other disciplines such as psychology, sociology, anthropology, philosophy, artificial intelligence, and communication science.

Within linguistics we can identify at least three views of how pragmatics relates to the other areas of language study. In the first view pragmatics is seen as the study of *language use*, while other areas of linguistics are concerned with *language structure*. A second view sees structure and use as distinct aspects of language that are related by pragmatics. In this view pragmatics explains the *relationship between language structure and language use*. Finally, there is a third view in which pragmatics is seen as an *area of language analogous to the other areas of language study* – phonology, syntax, and semantics. In this view similar principles and rules of organization which are to be found in phonology, syntax and semantics are also to be found in pragmatics. These three views of pragmatics are discussed in greater detail in this chapter, and in Chapter 2 other approaches to the study of language usage are examined that have been found to be relevant to an understanding of pragmatic disability.

Pragmatics as the study of language use

In this view of pragmatics, a distinction is made between the study of the structure of language and the study of the use of language. The traditional areas of linguistics – phonology, syntax, and semantics – are concerned with structure, while the use of these structures is the concern of pragmatics. This view can be represented diagrammatically, as in Figure 1.1.

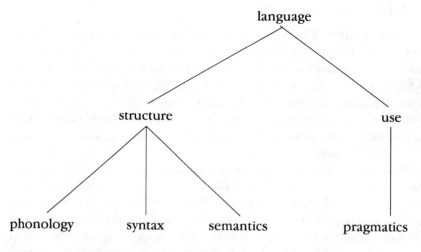

Figure 1.1 Pragmatics in the use of language

What are the aspects of language use that are the concern of pragmatics under this view? Taking a broad perspective, we might wish to assign to pragmatics anything that cannot be handled within phonology, syntax and semantics. Pragmatics would then be the study of language performance, which would include questions such as: How do we process sentences? How do we produce sentences? How does context help us determine the meaning of ambiguous sentences? What is involved in producing sentences that are appropriate in the contexts in which they are used? In other words, pragmatics is the study of all those aspects of language that have little or nothing to do with language structure but that have a bearing on how we use language in context.

One advantage of this view is that greater emphasis is placed on the study of the use of language. Traditionally there has been greater emphasis on studying language structure – possibly because language structure seemed to be more amenable to analysis. However, it is clear that anyone who has an interest in how language is used – including teachers, speech–language pathologist, and students of communication – must also be concerned with the systematic study of language usage. Thus the development of a theory of language usage is as important as the development of a theory of language structure.

There is a danger, however, of simply calling everything "pragmatic" that we cannot describe in more traditional terms. This approach has been referred to as the "pragmatic wastebasket". Clearly there is a need to bring some order into this wastebasket. Furthermore, it will be necessary to distinguish pragmatics from other branches of linguistics that are also concerned with the study of language usage. For example, the study of psychological aspects of language usage, such as linguistic perception and processing, overlaps with the field of psycholinguistics, while the study of social aspects of language usage overlaps with sociolinguistics.

More positively, we can identify several areas within the study of language usage that may be seen as relatively independent of the study of structure. These are: language as social action, language as appropriate behavior, and language as a means of intentional communication.

Language as social action
Language as social action is concerned with the study of linguistic acts in social contexts. As Green (1989, p.3) writes: "The broadest interpretation of pragmatics is that it is the study of understanding intentional human action." To understand intentional human action we need to study the nature of intentions, beliefs, wishes, and plans. For example, if we want to convince someone that we like him or her, we will have an intention to do or say something that will achieve this effect, which may involve developing a plan of action in which we try to change that person's current beliefs. If we want to tell a lie, we must say something that we

believe to be untrue but we must get our hearer to believe that we actually believe it is true. However, if we tell a joke, then we may also say something that we believe to be untrue but we will also want the hearer to see that we believe it is untrue.

Social actions such as these which involve the use of language have been referred to as speech acts. Speech acts are one of the most widely studied phenomena in pragmatics. Put simply, a speech act is the social action that is accomplished through the use of language. For example, in performing a particular utterance in a certain way and in a certain context we may be making a promise, issuing a threat, asking a question, paying a compliment, and so on. Speech acts have been used widely as a basic concept in the study of child language acquisition, second language learning, literary criticism, computational linguistics, and, more recently, speech–language pathology. We will look at speech acts in greater detail in Chapter 2 and examine the acquisition of the ability to use speech acts in Chapter 4.

Language as appropriate behavior
While there are many different ways to ask someone to close the door, it is usually the case that not all of the theoretically possible forms are appropriate in a particular context. Some of the forms are more polite than others and in some contexts a more polite form would be more appropriate. Some forms are also more indirect than others. Similarly, there are contexts in which an indirect form is more appropriate than a direct form.

What do we mean by context? Context is a difficult term to define. In a broad sense we might include all the features of a situation that are relevant to how an utterance is produced and understood. These might include: the roles and status of the speakers; the time and place of the utterance; and the subject matter of the utterance. So, to take a simple example, the form of a request will vary according to the roles and status of the speaker and addressee as well as to the nature of what is being requested. Accordingly, a person of subordinate status addressing a superior would be likely to choose a more polite form of request, while a superior addressing a subordinate is not required to show deference in this way. Similarly, if the object of the request is something simple, such as asking for a match, then an elaborate form is unnecessary, whereas a request that places greater demands on the addressee, such as asking for some special favor, is more appropriately couched in a form that reflects deference and consideration.

It is clear that with the terms "context" and "appropriacy" we are addressing two concepts in pragmatics that lie outside the concerns of the study of language structure but are central to the study of language use. While we can study the structure and meaning of sentences independently of their use, as soon as we wish to analyze why a particular sentence is used or why a sentence, which out of context is ambiguous but in context has only one meaning, then we need to evoke these concepts. This is not to say that the analysis of language usage becomes straightforward. Specifying those features that are culturally and linguistically relevant to the production and interpretation of utterances is a major research activity in pragmatics, which overlaps with and draws on many of the concerns of sociolinguistics. Moreover, judgments of appropriacy are not categorical in the way that judgments of grammaticality are. By this we mean that, while in many cases there is general agreement about what linguistic behavior is appropriate in a given context, our judgments are relative. There are degrees of appropriacy to a much greater extent than there are degrees of grammaticality. As well as this, people often adopt apparently inappropriate behaviors as a strategic resource. For example, a person may be intentionally rude if this seems to be the best way of achieving a particular goal.

In addition to the notions of context and appropriacy, there has been considerable interest in pragmatics in describing the general principles that guide the conduct of conversation. The best known example was developed by the philosopher Grice who identified four basic maxims of conversation which together contribute to a more general cooperative principle that underlies conversational participation (Grice, 1975). The cooperative principle states generally that participants should produce utterances that contribute to the purposes and direction of the conversation. This does not, of course, mean that they should always agree or comply with each other's demands, but that they should say things that are relevant, true, informative, and clear – requirements that are specified in the four basic maxims of conversation. Once again these are principles that are concerned with the ways in which language is used and that can be formulated independently of considerations of language structure. It will soon become apparent, however, how Grice's principles were intended to be more than a set of prescriptive rules for how conversation ought to be and how they can be used to explain a crucial phenomenon in pragmatics – how utterances can be taken to mean something over and above what they mean on a literal reading.

Language as a means of intentional communication
Language has been described as the primary means that humans use to communicate. Clearly there are also nonlinguistic means of communication that can be used effectively, such as shaking a fist to make a threat or waving to greet. Moreover, there is a whole range of nonverbal behavior that accompanies linguistic communication, such as posture, proximity to the hearer, hand movements, and eye gaze (see Ellis and Beattie (1986) for a recent discussion). However, in addition to a description of these various means of communication and how they are

used, a definition is required of what communication is.

Communication has often been defined in terms of the transmission of a message between a sender and a receiver. This definition is insufficient because it fails to distinguish between information that is involuntarily or unconsciously conveyed and information that is intentionally communicated. For example, a mother might infer that her baby is hungry because the baby is crying in a particular way, but we cannot conclude that the baby has intended to communicate through its crying that it is hungry. Similarly, a person might move a hand in a particular gesture without meaning to convey anything in particular with that hand movement. For this reason it is necessary to include intention in a definition of communication.

However, it has been argued that human communication requires more than the intention to communicate a message. As Grice (1968) has shown, the sender must not only intend to communicate a message, but should understand that the receiver is able to recognize that intention. Without this condition many attempts at communication would be doomed to failure. For example, it would be pointless trying to communicate a complex piece of information in French to someone who is known not to speak French, because it will be clear to the sender that the receiver will not be able to recognize the sender's intention (except, perhaps, that the sender is trying to communicate something).

Finally, the sender needs to recognize that the receiver is an independent agent with goals and beliefs that are to be distinguished from those of the sender. Accordingly, the receiver may understand what the sender intends to communicate and may indicate to the sender that this intention has been recognized, without necessarily complying with the demands of the sender's message.

To bring these points together: we have defined communication as involving:

- an intention to communicate some information to another person;
- the understanding that successful communication requires that the other person should be able to recognize that intention to communicate;
- the recognition that the other person, while recognizing the sender's communicative intentions, may have goals and beliefs that are different from those of the sender.

In Chapter 4 it will become obvious how this definition of communication is crucial to an analysis of early communicative behaviors in babies and infants; it will also be important in the examination of children's ability to assess the intentions and beliefs of other persons when the development of a theory of mind in children is examined (see Chapter 6).

Pragmatics as relating language form and language use

We have seen how pragmatics can be viewed as the study of language usage more or less independently of the study of how language is structured. Speech acts, context, appropriacy, conversational maxims, and our definition of intentional communication were examples of this view of pragmatics. However, we often need to explain aspects of language use in terms of the linguistic forms used or, conversely, to explain why particular linguistic forms are chosen rather than others in terms of pragmatic considerations. Accordingly, it is possible to identify a second view in which pragmatics is seen as being concerned with rules and principles that relate the structure of language to its use. This view can be represented as in Figure 1.2.

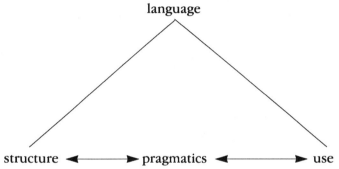

Figure 1.2 Pragmatics as relating language structure and language use

Here some examples of these rules and principles are examined.

Speech acts

Earlier speech acts were introduced as linguistic expressions that are used to achieve particular effects in social contexts and a distinction was made between speech acts in terms of speaker's and hearer's beliefs and intentions. It was also indicated that there are certain conditions that must be fulfilled for a speech act to be performed appropriately. These aspects of speech acts can be discussed independently of considerations of language structure.

However, if speech acts are examined in greater detail, usually they cannot be analyzed independently of language form. To take a simple example: there are many different ways of asking someone to close the door, such as:

1. Close the door.
2. Would you close the door?
3. I'd appreciate if you would close the door.
4. Is that door open?
5. There's a draught in here.

While each of these sentences may be uttered in order to perform the speech act of asking the hearer to close the door, they clearly use different words and different grammatical forms which have a bearing on the degree of politeness of the request as well as on the degree of directness with which it is expressed. Thus it is necessary to explain how the choice of particular linguistic forms relates to the particular speech act that is being performed, and, more problematically, how a sentence such as "There's a draught in here" can have a literal meaning as well as an indirect meaning *(close the door)* and how people can use and understand these meanings effortlessly in everyday conversation. Much effort has been expended in the attempt to answer questions such as these in speech act theory, although no entirely satisfactory solutions have been proposed. Although speech acts can be viewed as an aspect of language use that can often be examined independently of language structure, there is an inevitable need to relate form and function when trying to explain how particular forms can be used to perform particular speech acts. These issues will be taken up in greater detail in Chapter 2.

Conversational maxims

The conversational maxims which Grice proposed could be seen as a prescriptive view of how conversation should be. It would then be possible to examine particular conversations for the extent to which they conform to the maxims. However, Grice intended the maxims to be understood in a more interesting way – to explain how utterances can mean (or *implicate*) something over and above their literal meanings. Thus the maxims can be used to explain occasions when speakers do not answer in the most obvious or direct way. To take an example:

    A: Where's the newspaper?
    B: Where's your glasses?

At first sight B's response seems inappropriate, because B answers with a question rather than saying where the newspaper is, which would be a more direct answer to the question. Thus B appears to be violating the maxims of relevance and quantity by saying something that does not seem to be relevant and that is not informative. However, it is not difficult to find an interpretation to B's answer if we take it at a deeper level and assume that B is intending to respond to A's question – in other words, B is cooperating in the conversation by saying something that contributes to the general purpose and direction of the conversation. Thus B might be suggesting the following: A has asked for the newspaper because he cannot see where it is; if A were wearing his glasses, he would be able to see where the newspaper is. Thus, by assuming that B is being cooperative at a deeper level, the connection between the two utterances can be seen.

More generally, the assumption that the cooperative principle is being adhered to despite superficial appearances allows participants in conversation to make inferences about what is meant which take us beyond the literal meaning of the utterances. These conversational inferences are examined in greater detail in Chapter 2.

Context and grammar
One important concern in pragmatics is to explain the use of particular linguistic forms in terms of their context of use. This aspect of pragmatics has been referred to as the "grammaticalization of context". A simple example is the use of address terms – for example, when to use first names, names with titles such as Mr, Mrs, Dr, or, as in many languages, different forms for the pronoun *you*.

More generally, the most obvious examples of the relationship between language and context are to be found in the study of *deixis*, which describes how languages encode features of the context of utterance. Examples are the differences between *this* and *that, come* and *go, here* and *there*. In each case the choice of the appropriate term depends on whose perspective is being taken – the speaker's or the listener's. For example, *come here* would normally mean "move in the direction of the speaker" while *go there* means "move in a direction away from the speaker". A further aspect of the use of deictic terms is that they cannot usually be understood outside the context in which they have been used. So, for example, a child speaking on the telephone and saying "I like this one" (while holding up a picture) will not be easily understood by the person at the other end of the line. Both aspects of deixis have been studied in child language research – the choice of the appropriate term and the ability to assess accurately the context in which the term can be used. The second of these is particularly important for assessing whether a child is able to adopt the listener's perspective in conversation.

Other examples of the grammaticalization of context involve functional explanations for linguistic facts. The choice between passive and active sentences has already been mentioned. Other examples include the use of cleft constructions ("It was Darren who broke the window" as opposed to "Darren broke the window"), as well as the encoding of given and new information – for example, when to use the definite article *(the)* as opposed to the indefinite article *(a)*. These choices depend, on the one hand, on what was previously said and how the current utterance relates to that, and on the other, on contextual considerations such as whether the listener can retrieve the item being referred to. The first set of conditions is linguistic because they deal with relationships between sentences that can be explained in linguistic terms; the second set of conditions is extralinguistic, because they refer to phenomena outside of language, such as the context of the utterance or the listener's knowledge.

It is important to consider the relationship between context and linguistic form, because the choice of a particular form often depends on the context in which it is used and children may often have difficulty in making an appropriate choice or in understanding the relevance of the choice of one form over another in speech addressed to them. The problem could be that, although they have command over the required linguistic forms, they do not understand the contexts in which it is appropriate to use these forms. This would be an example of a pragmatic difficulty, even though what is involved is the use (or nonuse) of a particular grammatical form. Difficulties in this area can impinge on social relations, in as much as they affect perceptions of politeness and appropriate behavior; they also affect comprehension of content, because the inability to specify accurately the referents of the discourse, or to retrieve those referenced in another's speech, can lead to confusion and misunderstanding.

Pragmatics as a level of linguistic analysis

The third view is that pragmatics is a level of linguistic analysis that can be distinguished from and defined in terms of other levels. This is the most controversial of the three views that have been identified here and it can be represented diagrammatically, as in Figure 1.3.

The arguments for or against pragmatics as a level of linguistic analysis are fairly technical and not particularly relevant to the analysis of pragmatic disability. For this reason some points in support of this view are only briefly mentioned here (for more detailed discussion, see Levinson, 1983; Stubbs, 1983).

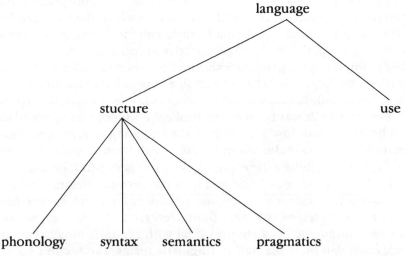

Figure 1.3 Pragmatics as a level of linguistic analysis

Pragmatics in relation to semantics
Earlier it was mentioned that semantics can be defined as the study of meaning. However, it is also possible to mean more than what is literally expressed by an utterance. For this reason, semantics has been more precisely defined as the study of conventional or literal meaning, while other meanings have been explained in terms of pragmatic phenomena, such as conversational inferences. The nature of these conversational inferences is examined in greater detail in Chapter 2.

Another aspect of language with which a semantic theory will have difficulty concerns the meanings of certain linguistic expressions, for example, simple conjunctions such as *and, if* and *because*. This can be illustrated with some examples.

Conjunctions seem to have more than one meaning. The literal meanings, which are the concern of a semantic theory, would be as follows:

and – joins together two independent clauses, e.g. snow is white and coal is black
if – relates a condition and a consequence, e.g. if you drink too much you will become ill
because – relates an effect and a cause, e.g. he went home because he felt ill

However, these conjunctions can be used with additional meanings, as follows:

he fell ill and died
(the clauses cannot be reversed, compared to the previous example, so that *and* has the additional meaning here of *and then*)
if you're hungry there's some cake in the fridge
(the presence of the cake does not depend on the addressee's hunger: the meaning is nonconventional and expresses an indirect offer)
he was drunk, because I saw him staggering
(seeing a person staggering does not cause him to be drunk: the meaning is one of assertion + justification).

Difficulties also occur with establishing the meanings of words and phrases (or particles) such as *well, anyway* and *by the way*, and adverbs such as *moreover* and *frankly*. Definitions for items such as these are not to be found in dictionaries because their meanings are defined in terms of their discourse functions. Examples include: one use of *well* is in a general introductory function, as in "Well, what do you think?", indicating a break in the discourse topic and signalling a new section of discourse. A second meaning occurs when *well* is used to preface an indirect answer to a question, as in:

A: Did you do the shopping?
B: Well, I ran into an old friend and ...

On hearing *well* it should be clear to A that B has not done the shopping as expected. The item *by the way* has the function of signalling a break in the topic, while *anyway* is used to indicate that the speaker wants to return to a previous topic, as in "Anyway, what do you think of my new suit?" (See Levinson (1983) and Stubbs (1983) for further examples and discussion involving other adverbs and particles.)

The structural analysis of discourse

"Discourse analysis" is a term used particularly in British linguistics to refer to the linguistic analysis of spoken and written discourse, where a discourse is taken to be a unit of analysis larger than the sentence – for example, a paragraph in written discourse, or in spoken discourse a speech event such as an interview or a conversation (Brown and Yule, 1983; Stubbs, 1983). Given that there are these larger units, it is interesting to examine the ways in which they are structured. A great deal of work has been done in this area, some of which will be dealt with again in Chapter 2. For the present, it will be helpful to introduce briefly the notion of conversational structure.

If any conversation is examined and a conversational turn is taken as a basic unit, then it will be clear that turns do not occur in isolation but are related to each other in sequences. To take a simple example: a first turn might ask a question while the next turn provides an answer. To put this another way: the first turn predicts a response, while the second turn provides the response. This structural principle, which forms the basis of the notion of the *adjacency pair*, applies to many other types of conversational turn, such as statement – acknowledgment, request – compliance, offer – acceptance, and compliment – acceptance. The structures are more complicated than suggested here, as will be shown in Chapter 2. Moreover, there have been alternative analyses of the structure of conversation, the most notable of these being the analysis of *exchange structure* in the approach known as Birmingham Discourse Analysis (see, for example, Stubbs, 1983; Coulthard, 1985). However, the main point is that a possible analogy can be drawn with other levels of linguistic analysis, in particular syntax. So, while in syntax it is possible to specify the ways in which units can be combined (for example, determiners precede nouns and, more generally, there are rules determining which combinations are well formed and which are not) likewise, it seems that similar principles of organization apply in conversation. If there is such a structure to conversation, then it will be important to investigate how and whether children acquire an ability to structure their conversations in accordance with these principles for well-formed conversations.

Which view of pragmatics is relevant for studying pragmatic disability?

Three views have been presented of how pragmatics might be defined within linguistic theory and the impression may have been given that these three views are incompatible. However, for practical purposes, when studying pragmatic disability, it will be helpful to be able to make use of all three views. At times there is a focus on principles of the use of language, such as speech acts, conversational maxims or intentional communication, without being concerned with linguistic structure. The reason for this is that children have to acquire these principles in order to communicate effectively and so it is proper to study the principles of language use in their own right. This allows the examination of cases of children who have little or no difficulty with language structure but who have problems in applying the principles of language use. However, it will also be important to examine the ways in which language structure and language use are related, and to do this it is necessary to adopt the second view in which the questions looked at include the relationship between the forms and functions of speech acts, the role of conversational maxims in generating conversational inferences, and the effects of context on grammatical structure. By taking this view light will be shed on those children whose problems lie in the interrelationships between language structure and language use. Finally, by adopting the third view it will be possible to investigate issues such as the relationship between conventional and nonconventional meaning that will help in understanding those children who have difficulty with this aspect of language use.

In sum, although three positions within linguistics have been identified regarding the definition of pragmatics, for practical purposes the distinctions are often blurred and it is a matter of emphasis when a decision is taken to adopt one view rather than another. Indeed, as shown in Chapter 2, it will be important to go beyond linguistic pragmatics to examine other approaches to the study of language use if we are to understand more fully what is involved in the acquisition of communicative competence by young children.

Pragmatics and speech–language pathology

In attempting to answer the question "What is pragmatics?", different views of the position of pragmatics in linguistic theory have been examined. Pragmatics can be described generally as the study of the rules governing the use of language in social contexts. Some examples were presented at the beginning of this chapter which illustrated some of the difficulties that children may have in the use of language. Pragmatic disability is examined in greater detail in Chapters 4, 5 and 6. However, it might be helpful at this point to indicate what is new about pragmatics and to review some reasons why it is important for speech–language pathologists to be concerned about pragmatics.

What is new about pragmatics?

It is legitimate for practitioners such as speech–language pathologists and teachers to argue that pragmatics is nothing new – they have always been concerned with how people might be helped to use language effectively in everyday communication and have developed practical procedures to help children who have difficulties in this aspect of language. That, after all, is what speech–language pathology and much of education is about. Indeed, it could be argued that, while research in pragmatics over the last 10 years or so marks a new approach within linguistic theory (or, more generally, the theory of communication), those working at the "front line" have been putting these ideas into practice using intuition, commonsense and experience to guide them. Now they are presented with what may appear to be no more than the ideas and principles that have formed the basis of their everyday practice, but dressed up in a complex, confusing, and sometimes impenetrable terminology. In other words, while theoretical linguists have been concerning themselves with questions such as the autonomy of syntax or the modularity of language, and ignoring questions concerning the use of language, practitioners have always maintained a more functional view of language as a tool for communication in everyday contexts.

Although the authors agree with the general drift of this viewpoint, it can be argued that recent developments in pragmatic theory have something to offer to the practitioner. In order to do this, it is necessary to sketch briefly the relationship between linguistic theory and speech–language pathology practice.

At the risk of over-simplification, it could be said that linguistic theory over the last three decades has focused on the study of syntax. Within this period debates have been concerned with delimiting the role of a semantic theory in relation to an autonomous syntax, and, more recently, with investigating the relationships between pragmatics and syntax, on the one hand, and pragmatics and semantics, on the other. In contrast, a view of speech–language pathology (again much over-simplified) shows a move away from an almost exclusive focus on problems of articulation to other levels of language: first syntax and lexical semantics, and, more recently, pragmatics. In other words, a close correlation does not always exist between developments in linguistic theory and developments in speech–language pathology practice. One possible conclusion could be that practitioners cannot allow themselves to be constrained by the theorists. After all, they have a job to do right now and cannot wait until the theorists come up with some ideas on how they should proceed. In any case, much of what is included under pragmatics would seem to be a matter of commonsense.

Although it is important to be continually aware of practical issues, it can be argued that theory is important and that considerable benefits can be derived from examining theoretical issues in linguistics and other disciplines, in as much as they impinge on our understanding of how language is used in communication. At the very least, work within a coherent and consistent framework is more likely to prevent the problems of theoretical and terminological confusion that currently pervade the study of pragmatic disability. On a more positive note, there should be a two-way communication between theory and practice, so that, for example, findings from the work of speech–language pathologists with "pragmatically disordered" patients would have an impact on pragmatic theory, while new insights from theory might help to put into a clearer perspective what might at first appear to be unrelated or unexplained phenomena.

Why pragmatics is important for speech–language pathologists

The usefulness of pragmatics to speech–language pathologists can be illustrated by drawing on a useful distinction between two different ways of viewing pragmatics in a speech–language pathology context. In this view pragmatics can be considered either as (1) a perspective on interpersonal and communicative approaches to language assessment and remediation or (2) as a way of focusing on a range of disabilities that lie beyond traditional areas of inquiry and which concern functional rather than structural aspects of language. These views have been referred to respectively as "broad pragmatics" and "narrow pragmatics" (Craig, 1983).

The term "broad pragmatics" emphasizes the need to consider the contextual aspects of communication. So, for example, one of the concerns of broad pragmatics might be the question of the extent to which a speech–language pathologist's therapeutic style has a bearing on the client's performance. Such questions have a long history and we can point to similar questions being asked in educational circles in work on classroom interaction analysis. Contextual issues are also brought to bear on assessment procedures, as seen, for example, in the concern in recent tests of pragmatic disability with devising procedures for the elicitation of a client's language which appear closer to the processes of naturally occurring conversation. These important issues will be returned to in later chapters, particularly in Chapters 7 and 8.

Another question concerns the everyday contexts in which children use language and the question of the extent to which deficiencies in the ability to use language effectively in communicative contexts affect their social relationships and development. In this respect it is possible to point to important studies of children's friendships in which the peer social world of childhood and the dynamic processes of friendship formation have been studied in detail (Gottman and Parker, 1986). Among the most relevant findings from the present perspective is one in which there appear to be differences in conversational skills between those children perceived by their peers as popular and those perceived as unpopular. For example, popular children used the strategy of trying to establish a common frame of reference with other group members in terms of activities and goals, while unpopular children tended to use the strategy of drawing attention to themselves. Popular children were also better at clarifying misunderstandings and resolving conflict, for example, by giving justifications or using polite strategies. Similarly, it has been reported that learning-disabled children are less popular in peer contexts because other children find difficulty in interacting with them (Donahue, 1987). Because some of these difficulties appear to involve communication skills, it seems appropriate that greater attention should be paid to the development of these skills in order to enhance the social well-being of these children. For these reasons it is important to examine the nature of clinician–child discourse, because this is the context in which the assessment and remediation of communication problems occurs. It is also necessary to compare this context with the everyday communicative situations in which the child is required to interact with other people. These issues are dealt with in greater detail in Chapter 8.

This brings us to the second view of pragmatics, which focuses on ways in which people might have a disability in some aspect of the use of language. In this "narrow" view of pragmatics the main concern is with an additional set of rules for using language that are distinct from rules of linguistic structure. Examples are turn-taking, producing and understanding speech acts such as requests and promises, telling stories, and repairing conversational breakdowns. Some examples were discussed earlier and these aspects of communication are examined in greater detail in Chapter 4. What is important for clinicians to note is that there is an additional set of skills that need to be assessed and trained. There is a need to be aware of the complex rules that children have to acquire in order to use language appropriately and effectively in a variety of contexts. There is also a need for more tools to help clinicians: to identify, in a principled way, those children who may have difficulties in the area of pragmatics; and to obtain intervention guidelines for remediation.

Concluding remarks

In this chapter the notion of pragmatic disability has been introduced. A start was made with some examples that illustrate the difficulties some children have in using language in everyday communication. Different views of pragmatics within linguistics were then examined and some of the key concepts outlined – these will be drawn on when pragmatic disability is examined. Among these concepts were: speech acts, appropriacy, intentional communication, conversational maxims, contextual influences on grammar, pragmatic aspects of meaning, and the structure of discourse. The relevance of pragmatics for speech–language pathologists was also looked at and the importance of a comprehensive theoretical framework was stressed within which pragmatic disability can be investigated and understood.

In the next chapter coverage of pragmatics and the study of language use are extended, starting with a more detailed account of key issues in linguistic pragmatics. These were only introduced briefly in this chapter. Finally some other approaches to the study of language use are examined which will inform the subsequent discussion of pragmatic disability.

Chapter 2
Pragmatics and the
Study of Language Use

In the previous chapter, three different views of pragmatics within linguistics were examined and a brief introduction provided to those aspects that are of most concern to speech–language pathologists investigating problems of language use. In this chapter, coverage of the study of language use is extended first of all by elaborating on those aspects of linguistic pragmatics that are fundamental for speech–language pathologists investigating the use of language: speech acts, pragmatic aspects of meaning, and conversational structure. Following this different approaches to the study of language use are examined in disciplines other than linguistics – cognitive psychology, conversational analysis, and artificial intelligence. The wider perspective adopted by examining the contributions of these other disciplines creates a better position for understanding and explaining the nature of pragmatic disability.

Linguistic pragmatics

Three different views of pragmatics were considered in Chapter 1 and the following issues which were introduced will now be expanded upon: speech acts, pragmatic aspects of meaning, and conversational structure.

It is worth noting in passing that some of the work to be discussed in this section also goes under the name of discourse analysis. As mentioned in Chapter 1, the term "discourse analysis" has been used particularly in British linguistics to refer to the linguistic analysis of spoken or written discourse (Brown and Yule, 1983; Stubbs, 1983). Several issues have been investigated within this perspective:

– differences in form between written and spoken language;
– the structure of spoken discourse;
– the role of context in interpretation;
– discourse as a level of linguistic analysis.

24

Some of these issues clearly overlap with those studied in pragmatics, so it is legitimate to ask whether discourse analysis and pragmatics are really just different names for the same thing. For those who wish to make a distinction, it might be helpful to view discourse analysis as being concerned with the linguistic analysis of relationships between spoken or written sentences, while pragmatics deals with the relationship between these sentences and the contexts in which they are used. In other words, the focus in discourse analysis is on the linguistic characteristics of texts (either oral or written), while pragmatics is concerned with extralinguistic factors, such as context, and how they affect language use. Of course, as with many distinctions this one is particularly blurred and in practice the terms are often used interchangeably.

Pragmatics and language as social action: speech acts

Speech act theory developed out of the concerns of philosophers of language, such as Wittgenstein, who claimed that utterances could only be explained in relation to the activities (or *language games*) in which they are used, and Austin, whose work *How to do Things with Words* introduced speech act theory. These early ideas were subsequently developed by the philosopher Searle.

One of the main concerns of speech act theory is to establish the conditions under which a speech act can be performed. These conditions, which have been referred to as *felicity* or *appropriacy conditions*, are distinct from considerations of grammatical structure. Consequently, we can distinguish between sentences that are ungrammatical, such as "He lives in the city since three years", which can nevertheless usually be understood in context, and sentences that are inappropriate, even though they may be grammatically well-formed. To take an example: suppose someone says "I'll buy you an ice cream tomorrow". For this utterance to be acceptable as a promise, several conditions have to be fulfilled, including:

1. The speaker has said he or she will do an action at some future time.
2. The speaker intends to do the action.
3. The speaker believes he or she can do the action.
4. The speaker would not have done the action in the normal course of events.
5. The speaker believes that the hearer wants him or her to do the action.
6. The speaker intends to be placed under an obligation to do the action having made this utterance.

We can see that violation of any of these conditions renders the utterance unacceptable as a promise. For example, a promise cannot refer to some past event (condition 1), the speaker must be sincere (condition 2), while if the speaker believes the hearer does not want the action, then the utterance may be a threat rather than a promise (condition 5). Similar conditions can be stated for other speech acts and it is possible to examine whether these conditions are applied in actual speech situations. For example, we can study the acquisition of children's use of speech acts (see, for example, Garvey, 1975; McTear, 1985a), or how language-disabled children have difficulty with particular aspects of speech act usage (see Chapter 4).

In addition to the question of the appropriacy of speech acts, there is the problem of working out what speech act is intended by an utterance, given that speakers may choose to express their intentions indirectly. For example: a speaker might say "It's cold in here", intending that the addressee should close the door. But how does the addressee come to infer this meaning, because the utterance might equally well have been used to suggest that "in here" is a good place to keep the beer cool, or indeed simply to mean what it expresses quite literally.

One explanation of how indirect meanings are resolved is in terms of specific rules of inference that allow us to derive the function (or force, as it is often referred to in speech act theory) of an utterance from its linguistic form and literal meaning. This can be illustrated by showing how such rules of inference have been used to explain how indirect requests are related to their linguistic forms.

The conditions that underlie the appropriate performance of speech acts have also been used to explain the basis for inferring the force of utterances. For example: Labov and Fanshel (1977) proposed conditions for requests, including: a need for the action, a need for the request, the hearer's ability, willingness and obligation to perform the action; the speaker's right to make the request. One rule of inference proposed by Labov and Fanshel is as follows:

> If a speaker makes an assertion or request for information about these conditions, then he can be heard as making a request for action. In addition, the speaker can also refer to the existential state of the action (whether it has been performed or not), the consequences of performing it, and the time when it might be performed.

Applying these rules, we can see how the following requests to dust a room can be related to the linguistic forms used to make the requests:

Existential status
Have you dusted yet?
You don't seem to have dusted this room yet.

Consequences
How would it look if you were to dust this room?
This room would look a lot better if you dusted it.

Time referents
When do you plan to dust?
I imagine you will be dusting this evening.

Need for the action
Don't you think the dust is pretty thick?
This place is really dusty.

Similarly, Labov and Fanshel show how the conditions can be used in putting off a request. To illustrate with a couple of examples:

Existential status
Isn't it dusted already?
I did dust it.

Need for action
It looks clean to me.
Doesn't it look clean to you?

The question of the relationship between form and function has not been resolved within pragmatics and many would argue that the rule-governed explanations proposed in speech act theory do not entirely explain the meanings or functions that utterances may have in particular contexts. This problem will be dealt with presently on examination of the contribution of conversation analysis.

Pragmatics and meaning

The relationship between pragmatics and meaning is probably one of the most important concerns of pragmatic theory. One of the major theoretical issues involves the borderline between semantics – traditionally the level of language concerned with meaning – and pragmatics. In fact, pragmatics has been defined as

the study of all those aspects of meaning not captured in a semantic theory (Levinson, 1983,p.12).

The problem then is to decide what aspects of meaning are covered in semantics. Given the wide range of semantic theories, this is no easy task and any attempt to draw a borderline will run into complex discussions about what kind of semantic theory is being adopted. This issue is beyond the scope of this book, so the most straightforward viewpoint is taken that semantics is concerned with those aspects of meaning that are conventional – for example, the literal meaning of words and sentences. Pragmatics, in contrast, is concerned with those aspects of additional meaning that can be read into sentences without actually being encoded in them. Thus pragmatics could include the use of irony and metaphor. More generally, however, the most widely studied kinds of meaning in pragmatics are those associated with *implicature* (or inference) and *presupposition*. As these concepts are central to linguistic pragmatics, they will require more extended discussion.

Conversational implicature
Introductory texts on pragmatics abound with examples of language use where it is impossible to make sense of an utterance without going beyond its literal meaning. The following is a typical example:

A: Would you lend me some money to buy a coffee?
B: It's not Christmas.

No semantic interpretation of B's utterance in terms of what it literally means would enable A to work out whether B will lend A some money, or indeed whether B is responding at all to the request rather than changing the topic. To make sense of B's utterance, A has to read some additional meaning into it. In other words, A has to make inferences about what B might mean.

The term "inference" is used in different ways in pragmatics, so it will be useful to make a distinction here before returning to the example. One use of inference is in logic, where an inference is a mechanism for deriving valid conclusions from a set of given assumptions. To take a simple example: from the assumptions (or premises):

If it has been raining, the ground will be wet.
It has been raining.

it can validly be concluded:

The ground will be wet.

This sort of inference is referred to as *deductive inference*. Deductive inference is based on specific rules of deduction that can be applied to any sets of propositions. The particular rule that is involved here is called *Modus Ponens*, and it can be represented more generally as follows:

If P then Q

<u>P   (given P)</u>

Q

The premises are: (1) *If P is true then Q is true*, and (2) *P is true*, where any proposition can stand for the symbols P and Q. Using Modus Ponens on these premises, it can be concluded (3) *Q is true*. This conclusion is guaranteed to be logically valid.

In contrast to deductive inferences such as Modus Ponens, the sort of inference that was illustrated earlier is not guaranteed to be logically valid. Returning to the example of A and B above, A might have concluded that B did not intend to give some money for coffee. However, B could have continued by saying "Oh well, I suppose you're a deserving case". In this situation, A's initial inference would have been wrong (depending, of course, on what inference was derived from B's second utterance). This type of inference can be referred to as a *conversational* or *pragmatic inference*. The main concerns of pragmatic theory regarding this type of inference are to:

- provide an explicit account of how it is possible to mean more than is said;
- propose general principles for cooperative interaction as an explanation of inferences.

Grice's conversational maxims were encountered earlier and to recap: Grice (1975) proposed a principle of cooperative conversation, which he formulated as follows:

> Make your contribution such as is required, at the stage at which it occurs, by the accepted purpose or direction of the talk exchange in which you are engaged.

Elaborating on this principle, Grice proposed *four maxims of conversation* – quantity, quality, relevance, and manner, as follows:

QUANTITY
1. Make your contribution as informative as is required for the current purposes of the exchange.
2. Do not make your contribution more informative than is required.

QUALITY
Try to make your contribution one that is true.
1. Do not say what you believe to be false.
2. Do not say that for which you lack adequate evidence.

RELATION
Be relevant.

MANNER
Be perspicuous:
1. Avoid obscurity of expression.
2. Avoid ambiguity.
3. Be brief.
4. Be orderly.

Grice then showed how these maxims could be used to explain how it is possible to mean (or implicate) more than what was said. The mechanism involved is referred to as *implicature*. There are two types of implicature: *conventional implicature* and *conversational implicature.* Each of these is illustrated in turn.

Conventional implicatures refer to meanings that can be attached to an utterance on the assumption that the maxims are being observed. This can be illustrated with reference to the maxim of quantity, which requires that a speaker should be informative – that is, say what is required but not more than is required. Thus a speaker who is observing the maxim of quantity and says "Walter has three children" will conventionally implicate "Walter has only three children". This is in spite of the fact that it would be logically compatible with the truth of the utterance "Walter has three children" if it were the case that Walter had, for example, five children. It would still be true that he had three children (and to prove this the speaker could list three of the children), although to say this would not be particularly helpful – indeed, it would be liable to mislead. The fact that it is difficult to entertain the logically valid interpretation indicates how pervasive the maxims are in everyday conversation. Thus, a speaker observing the maxim of quantity would say no more and no less than was necessary for the listener to make the appropriate inference, providing the listener was operating under the assumption that the speaker was being cooperative in this way. Clearly it is part of a person's competence to be able to derive these "extra" meanings over and above the literal meanings of an utterance. The argument from pragmatic theory is that the ability to do so depends on a knowledge of the principles of cooperative communication. Similar examples can be provided for conventional implicatures that can be derived from the other maxims (see Levinson, 1983, pp. 105–109).

The second way in which the maxims can be used is to generate *conversational implicatures*. In this case the maxims are blatantly flouted (or exploited) for some communicative purpose. To illustrate how maxims can be flouted, look again at an earlier example:

A: Would you lend me some money to buy a coffee?
B: It's not Christmas.

In this example it appears that B is not following the maxim of relevance, because what B says does not appear to be relevant to A's request. However, if it is assumed by both speakers that B is still being cooperative (in a much less direct manner), then A can conclude that B's utterance means more than what it appears to mean and can engage in a process of inferencing to work out what B might have meant. In this case, A would have to rely on wide-ranging extralinguistic knowledge – for example, that at Christmas people give presents to each other. Conversational implicature is a very important aspect of communicative competence because people often use indirectness for a variety of strategic ends, for example, to soften a request. Similarly it is essential that the hearer should be able to make appropriate inferences in order to be able to derive the meaning of what has been implicated. An inability to go beyond the literal meanings of utterances and thus engage in conversational inferencing is a serious handicap in everyday communication.

This overview of implicatures is concluded by an indication of some of their distinguishing characteristics. The most important of these is that they are *defeasible* (or cancellable). In other words, it is possible to cancel the pragmatic inference by saying something more (by adding an additional premise). In the case of the utterance "Walter has three children" and the implicature "Walter has only three children", the implicature would be cancelled if the speaker were to have continued: "Walter has three children, and maybe more". In contrast, deductive (i.e. logical) inferences are not defeasible.

A second characteristic of implicatures is that they are *nondetachable* – that is, they are attached to the semantic content of what is said rather than to the linguistic form. Thus any utterance that means roughly the same as another utterance, regardless of its actual linguistic form, can give rise to the same conversational implicature.

Furthermore, implicatures are *calculable, nonconventional,* and *indeterminate*. Implicatures are calculable on the basis of principles of cooperative conversation, and the use of the maxims, as we have shown; they are nonconventional in that they go beyond the literal meaning of what is said; and they are indeterminate because the same words can be given different meanings on different occasions. Taken together, these characteristics indicate some of the complexities that confront a child using language to engage in communicative interaction.

Presupposition

The term "presupposition" is often used loosely in pragmatics to refer to the background assumptions against which an utterance, action, or idea makes sense. For example: "Fixing cars presupposes some knowledge of car mechanics." Presupposition has also been used in some child language studies to refer to assumptions made about the beliefs and intentions of other people. Used in these ways presupposition means roughly the same as *pragmatic context*.

In pragmatic theory, however, the term has a narrower meaning, referring to inferences or assumptions that are built into linguistic expressions. So, for example, there are implicative verbs such as *manage* and *forget* which trigger particular inferences, as in these examples:

John managed to stop in time
(presupposes) John tried to stop in time

John forgot to buy the sausages
(presupposes) John intended to buy (ought to have bought) the sausages

Definite descriptions also give rise to presuppositions. A definite description is an expression such as *the king*. If we say something like "The king has decided to abdicate", then we are presupposing that a king exists. Young children often have difficulty with such presuppositions when they assume that the presuppositions of what they say are shared with those of their listener. For example, a child might say "The cat has been run over", which presupposes that there was a cat (perhaps in the family), but the listener may not have been aware of this and may respond "What cat?"

Change-of-state verbs are also presupposition triggers, as in the well-known example "Have you stopped beating your wife?", which presupposes that the person addressed did at one time beat his wife. Similarly, there is a class of verbs, called factive verbs, that presuppose the truth of their complements. For example, the verbs *regret* and *realize* presuppose that the information stated in the following *that* clause is true, as in these examples:

> John realized that he had failed the exam
> (presupposes) John failed the exam
>
> Bill regretted that he had sold the car
> (presupposes) Bill sold the car

In contrast, nonfactive verbs do not behave in this way, as in this example:

> Stanley believed that he had won a prize
> (does not presuppose) Stanley won a prize

Indeed, there is a fairly definitive set of linguistic constructions that act as presupposition triggers in this way (Levinson, 1983, pp.181–184, mentions a list of 31 such triggers and gives examples of a selection of these). Someone who is competent in a language will be able to make the inferences that are built into and triggered by these constructions. As with implicatures, presuppositions give rise to inferences that allow speakers to mean more and hearers to understand more than what is literally said. Some research will be examined in Chapter 4 that has investigated children's ability to make judgments about the assumptions triggered by constructions such as these.

Presuppositions have one further important characteristic – *constancy under negation*. What this means quite simply is that the inferences triggered by a sentence will remain true even if the sentence is negated – as long as the inference is a presupposition. To illustrate:

> John managed to stop in time
> >> John stopped in time
> >> John tried to stop in time

Both sentences indicated with >> are inferences, but only the second holds up if we negate the sentence:

> John didn't manage to stop in time
> >> John tried to stop in time
> (but does not imply) John stopped in time

Presuppositions are like implicatures in that they are *defeasible* in certain contexts, that is, the inferences that they give rise true to are not necessarily true and can be cancelled by what is said subsequently. In the example discussed above, it would be possible to continue as follows:

John didn't manage to stop in time, in fact he didn't even try

In this case the presupposition that *John tried to stop in time* would be cancelled by the continuation *in fact he didn't even try*.

There are many more complex issues involving presupposition that would go beyond the scope of the present discussion. What has been presented will help readers understand the issues that have been investigated in children's understanding of presupposition, and are discussed in Chapter 4. Readers interested in more detailed discussion are referred to Levinson (1983, Chapter 4).

The structure of conversation

In Chapter 1 the notion of conversational structure was introduced and it was noted that utterances in conversation do not occur randomly but in some sort of sequence: questions are usually followed by answers, offers by acceptances or rejections, and requests by compliant actions or refusals. Two types of structural unit proposed for conversation are discussed: adjacency pairs and exchange structure.

Adjacency pairs

Adjacency pairs were proposed by a group known as Conversation Analysts (see below) to capture the notion that utterances often come in pairs (Schegloff and Sacks, 1973). For example: greeting–greeting; question – answer; offer–acceptance/refusal. Often more than one response is possible, as has been indicated in the case of responses to offers. Moreover, there can also be items embedded or inserted into an adjacency pair, as in this example:

A:	Have you seen Mary?	Question 1
B:	Mary who?	Question 2
A:	Mary Webster	Answer 2
B:	Oh her, no I haven't.	Answer 1

Similarly, some utterances seem to have a preparatory function in that they prepare the way for a subsequent pair of utterances:

A: Are you doing anything tonight?
B: No.
A: Well then, would you like to go out for a drink?
B: Sure.

If the third and fourth turns in this sequence are interpreted as an invitation and an acceptance, then the first and second turns can be viewed not as an independent question–answer pair but as a presequence – in this case, a preinvitation. Presequences often serve a strategic function because they allow a speaker to check the most probable grounds for failure of a subsequent utterance such as an invitation or a request and allow that sequence to be aborted, thus preventing loss of face by either participant.

Adjacency pairs also provide evidence of the conversational work involved in everyday talk. Speakers display their understandings of previous talk in their own utterances. For example, a response to a question can be inspected by the questioner to see whether the question has been understood or not. Thus speakers in a conversation are in a continuous process of monitoring each other's utterances within the predictions set up by preceding utterances, and are continually displaying to each other their understanding of these utterances.

Exchange structure
The exchange appears to be similar to the adjacency pair in that it is the minimal unit of interaction, consisting of at least one move by one speaker which *initiates* the exchange, and a second move by another speaker which *responds* to the exchange. Exchanges are part of a descriptive framework for the linguistic analysis of discourse developed by a group known as the Birmingham Discourse Analysts (Sinclair and Coulthard, 1975; Coulthard, 1985). The main aim of this work was to describe the structure of discourse events such as teacher–pupil interaction in classrooms. In this type of discourse it was found that exchanges often consisted of three parts in which the teacher asked a question with the purpose of eliciting a response, the pupil responded, and the teacher followed the response by accepting or evaluating it, before going on to another elicitation which would begin a further exchange. This structure has become known as initiation–response–feedback (IRF) and has also been found to occur frequently in talk between speech–language pathologist and their clients. The following is an example from classroom discourse:

Teacher:	What is the capital of France?	I	
Pupil:	Paris.	R	Exchange 1
Teacher:	Good.	F	
	And what is the capital of Italy?	I	
Pupil:	Naples.	R	Exchange 2
Teacher:	No.	F	

The first IRF sequence is part of exchange 1 and the second IRF sequence is part of exchange 2. It should also be noted that exchanges may cut across a speaker's turns. Thus the teacher's second turn consists of an F, which is part of exchange 1, and an I, which is part of exchange 2. Thus turns are not the relevant units in exchange structure, but rather *moves*. Furthermore, a move may be broken down into *acts*, as in the following example of an initiating move:

Teacher:	What about this one?	Starter
	This I think is a super one.	Starter
	Isobel.	Nomination
	Can you think what it means?	Elicitation

Here the teacher's initiating move consists of four acts: two starters, which prepare for the main act in the move, a nominating act, and then an eliciting act which is the main or head act.

Exchanges are similar to adjacency pairs in several ways. In exchanges, utterances can be *prospective*: that is, they set up constraints or expectations on a following utterance. They can also be *retrospective*, in that they fulfil the predictions of a previous utterance. However, there are also some differences. The Birmingham Discourse Analysts, starting from the aim of extending linguistic analysis beyond the level of the sentence, were interested in specifying the structure of discourse in terms of a hierarchy of units and rules for the combination of these units. Thus a discourse unit such as a lesson could be broken down into a series of smaller units called transactions, which could be broken down into exchanges. Exchanges consisted of moves and moves of acts. Furthermore, within units such as exchanges there was an ordering of items, so that initiations preceded responses. Similarly, within moves a nomination might precede an elicitation. Thus an analogy was drawn with syntactic analysis in which items were viewed in terms of constituency – sentences consist of phrases which consist of words – and ordering – determiners precede nouns, auxiliary verbs have a fixed ordering.

However, while this approach brought some rigor to the analysis of spoken and written discourse, it also resulted in many problems. One major difficulty was that this scheme of analysis did not seem to be easily applicable to casual conversation, because often utterances did not seem to be classifiable in terms of the more structured combinations that had been found in classroom talk. Although many attempts were made at providing alternative frameworks which might account for the structure of conversation, some felt that the attempt to push the analogy with syntactic analysis was misguided. In particular, the question arose as to whether there are in fact rules for well-formed conversations. An alternative approach will be examined in the next section. Finally, there was the criticism that this approach seemed to be too descriptive, focusing on the classification and labelling of utterances in a conversation and disregarding the interactional processes involved in conversation. (For a more detailed discussion of these issues, see Levinson, 1983, Chapter 6.)

Conversation analysis

Conversation analysis (or CA, as it is often called) is an empirical approach to conversation which studies the techniques used by conversationalists to interpret and act within a social world. Conversation analysis emerged out of the work of a breakaway group from traditional sociology known as *ethnomethodology*.

Workers in CA have investigated a wide range of conversational phenomena, such as turn-taking, adjacency pair structures, repair organization, providing, in each case, detailed descriptions based on careful analysis of naturally occurring data. Some of the findings of CA provide a useful basis for the investigation of the question of how people engage in everyday conversation (for a clear summary of the CA approach, see Levinson, 1983, Chapter 6). For example, some relevant questions are:

- How is turn-taking regulated in conversation? How do people know when to take a turn? What do they do when their talk overlaps?
- How do people respond to utterances such as questions, requests, invitations, compliments? What are the implications of the choice of a particular type of response?
- How are conversations organized as a whole and how do conversational participants collaborate to make conversations work?
- How do conversations break down and what strategies are used to repair these breakdowns?

These features have found their way into most of the checklists and similar procedures currently used for assessing pragmatic ability and will be examined in greater detail when dealing with the acquisition of conversational competence as well as pragmatic disability and its assessment in later chapters. For the present, it will be useful to highlight some general principles that have emerged from CA work and that distinguish this approach from the linguistic analysis of conversational structure described earlier.

Conversation as an interactional achievement

Conversation analysts emphasise that conversation is an interactional achievement. What they mean by this is that what emerges as a conversation is a product of the collaborative work of the participants in the conversation. Furthermore, the units of a conversation, such as utterances or turns, cannot be interpreted in isolation but only in relation to the overall context in which they occurred – what CA workers refer to as the sequential location of the utterance.

This emphasis on the interactional processes of conversation is important when we come to analyze conversations involving young children or children with pragmatic difficulties. There is a danger when analysing such conversations that the conversations are treated as a *product* rather than a *process*. In other words, the turns of each of the participants are coded – for example, as speech acts – and the analysis proceeds by determining whether the correct sequence of acts has been produced. In this way, it is possible to draw certain conclusions, such as attributing "blame" for conversational breakdown by indicating how a particular act was inappropriate.

The alternative approach, advocated in CA, is to determine the processes that have resulted in a particular conversational sequence. Thus how one person responds is influenced by the type of utterance to which the response is directed. To take a simple example: a child might fail to give the expected answer to a question, but the problem might lie in the question that was asked rather than in any inability or "blame" to be attributed to the child. In this view both participants collaborate as they engage in conversation and it is not possible to consider the contribution of one participant without considering what the other has said. This does not mean, however, that the participants must cooperate with each other in the sense of being compliant. What is meant, rather, is that no one participant can determine how the conversation will proceed and that what emerges is the outcome of an interaction between the participants.

A related notion is that utterances are not interpreted in isolation, but rather in relation to their sequential location. Thus what a particular utterance means is determined not by its linguistic properties alone, but by where it occurs in the conversation. This point is important in the analysis of a conversation because it is suggested that it is not possible to determine the functions of an utterance by simply examining its form. The classic discussion of this issue can be found in a paper by Schegloff (1978) where it is argued that an utterance such as "For whom?", which taken out of context would be interpreted as a question, in the particular context in which it was used was intended to express an entirely different function – to indicate agreement with the other speaker. As Schegloff describes in some detail, how the utterance can come to have this meaning is a function of its sequential location in the particular discourse in which it occurred.

Conversational structure

Conversation analysts have provided detailed analyses of conversational structure. *Adjacency pairs* have already been encountered – these capture the notion that utterances often come in pairs, for example, a question is often followed by an answer. The notion of exchange in linguistic discourse analysis was also discussed and this appears to address the same issue. However, as CA workers emphasize, conversational structure does not work in the same way as the rules of linguistics. To break a rule in syntax results in an ill-formed sentence; however, to break a rule in conversation does not result in an ill-formed conversation. Instead what happens is that a failure to follow an expected procedure gives rise to certain inferences – for example, a failure to respond to a greeting may be interpreted as a rebuff, while a failure to respond to a question may be interpreted as uncooperativeness or disagreement.

To see this point more clearly, we can consider what is involved in making a response to a previous utterance. It is often the case that more than one type of response is appropriate. For example, a response to a request might be to comply, but a person could also refuse, or could try to postpone compliance, or provide a reason for not complying. Thus there is often a range of alternatives from which a person might select. However, these alternatives do not have equal status. Some responses are classified in CA as *preferred* and others as *dispreferred*. Preference as used in CA does not refer to the preferences of the speakers in choosing what to say, but rather to differences between the choices they make. A preferred utterance is one which is unmarked or neutral, both in terms of its linguistic characteristics as well as the inferences it can give rise to. It will help to look at some examples.

Below two invitation sequences are examined (taken from Atkinson and Drew, 1979, p.58). In the first example, B responds with an acceptance, which is the preferred response:

A: Why don't you come up and see me some times?
B: I would like to.

In this example B responds affirmatively and without delay – in fact, the notation indicates that the beginning of B's utterance overlaps with the end of A's. Furthermore, B's response is simple and direct. In other words, in an invitation sequence an acceptance is the *preferred* response.

Consider, however, the following sequence in which B produces a *dispreferred* response – a rejection:

A: Uh if you'd care to come up and visit a little while this morning I'll give you a cup of coffee.

B: Hehh   well that's   awfully sweet of you.
        (DELAY)   (MARKER)   (APPRECIATION)
        I don't think I can make it this morning.
        (REFUSAL)
        Hh uhm I'm running an ad in the paper and uh I have to stay near
        the phone.
        (ACCOUNT)

Dispreferred responses are characterized by a number of features, as indicated in this example. Often the speaker will delay, either by pausing before responding or using hesitation markers, such as *hehh* or *uhm*. The response is often preceded by a word such as *well* which marks the response as dispreferred. In fact, *well* on its own would be sufficient to trigger the inference that B is not going to accept the invitation. A further feature is that the refusal may be mitigated, as in this example, whereas acceptances are usually simple and direct. Refusals are also often accompanied by an account.

The power of these features of dispreferred turns, such as delays in responding, can be seen in the following example taken from Levinson (1983, p. 320):

A: So I was wondering would you be in your office on Monday by any
        chance.
        (2.0)
        Probably not.
B: Hmm yes.

In this example A asks B a question. There is a 2-second pause, following which A continues *probably not*. Thus this brief delay in B's response has been sufficient to trigger the inference that B's response is negative – in other words, it is dispreferred. As it turns out, A has actually made the wrong inference as B goes on to reply in the affirmative, indicating that these inferences are defeasible.

More generally, it seems that there are often three classes of response to an utterance: the preferred response, a set of dispreferred responses, and a response (perhaps a silent response) in which no mention is made of either alternative. Thus it is possible to explain the inferences that arise when a person apparently fails to respond to a prior utterance – whether deliberately or not (Bilmes, 1988). For example, as seen previously, a person can accept or reject an invitation. But what happens if the response seems to be neither an acceptance nor a rejection? According to Bilmes, such a response gives rise to the inference that a rejection is intended. In other words, the schema for invitations sequences is as follows, where X represents a preferred response, Y a dispreferred response, and N represents no mention of either X or Y:

Invitation
X   Accept
Y   Refuse
N   No mention of X or Y
Inference: If N, then assume refusal

To explain: the preferred response to an invitation is to accept and the dispreferred response is to refuse. If no mention is made of either, the inference can be made that the response is a refusal.

This structure applies to other sequences such as requests or accusations. The following schema illustrates an accusation sequence:

Accusation
X   Denial
Y   Acceptance
N   No mention of X or Y
Inference: If N, assume acceptance of accusation

This sequence applies in everyday conversation but has also been adopted in some legal systems where a failure to respond in court is taken as an admission of guilt.

A final point about preference organization is that it can be used to explain various conversational phenomena in terms of speakers attempting to avoid the occurrence of dispreferred responses. Thus speakers will often precede a request with an utterance that "tests the water" such as "Are you busy at the moment?". Such pre-requests (or more generally, pre-sequences) serve the purpose of avoiding potential loss of face for one or both participants as the addressee can indicate whether the anticipated request is likely to be rejected, thus permitting the speaker to abandon the request and so avoid a dispreferred response. Thus indirect speech acts and hesitations can be explained as indications that a dispreferred response is anticipated in the next turn.

Summary

Conversation analysts have provided detailed analyses of conversation which enhance our understanding of how conversation works. In particular, they have provided a different perspective on conversational rules, which, rather than being viewed as a basis for judgments of well-formed discourse sequences, are seen as a basis for the interpretative procedures used by conversationalists to negotiate meanings and make inferences. These insights and principles are invaluable for those interested in the mechanisms of conversational interaction. They also indicate that certain approaches adopted in the analysis of conversation – such as counting the number of occurrences of particular types of conversational act – are ill-founded because they often fail to consider the interactional processes involved, the sequential location of the utterances, and the interpretative procedures and strategies applied by the participants in the conversation.

Psychological approaches to the study of language use

Many of the issues studied in linguistic pragmatics and conversation analysis are also investigated by psychologists – usually under the guise of discourse, text, interaction, or communication. Psychologists typically adopt a different approach to those described so far. In general, psychological investigations of pragmatics take the form of quantitative, experimentally based studies, in which usually some variable is isolated to test whether it influences the comprehension or production of language. Examples are the effects of pictures on the ability to comprehend and remember a story, the effects of eye-contact on turn-taking, or the question of whether listeners require greater processing time to understand indirect requests as opposed to direct requests. Thus studies have tended to be concerned with the degree of accuracy of recall or comprehension, or, in the case of reaction-time experiments, with comparisons of processing time under different conditions.

Other work has attempted to demonstrate that hearers use bridging inferences to make sense of sentences in a text which are not related explicitly. For example, consider what is involved in understanding the connection between the following two pairs of sentences, and, in particular, how to locate the definite expression, *the beer*:

Mary took the beer out of the car.
The beer was warm.

Mary took the picnic supplies out of the car.
The beer was warm.

Both pairs have identical second sentences. However, it would probably be more difficult to form a connection between the sentences in the second pair as there is no explicit prior mention of *the beer*. What is required to make this connection is a bridging inference, for example, that the picnic supplies included beer. In studies of listeners' reaction times to pairs of sentences such as these it was found that determining the referent (i.e. of *the beer*) in the second set took significantly longer than in the first set (Haviland and Clark, 1974). The implication is that making inferences takes time. A further important implication is that the ability to make inferences depends on background knowledge of the everyday world – for example, in this case that beer might be a part of the picnic supplies. This finding has led psychologists to investigate the psychological reality of knowledge structures and their role in text comprehension and production. This work derives in large part from research in artificial intelligence, which will be described in the next section. (For further discussion of psychologically based work on discourse, see Garnham, 1985, Chapter 7.)

The main strength of psychological studies of pragmatic issues is that they provide a methodology in which the relevant factors can be isolated and experimentally manipulated. Naturalistic studies suffer from the disadvantage that they are based on whatever data happen to present themselves. There is always the danger that any findings are a consequence of sampling bias and that they are not generalizable to other data. By controlling the relevant factors and by measuring effects using well-established experimental procedures, psychologists are able to test hypotheses about the nature of language use and provide statistically reliable results.

However, psychological approaches to pragmatics display several shortcomings. Experimental studies can be criticized for attempting to study natural conversation in artificially controlled environments. In order to permit sufficient experimental control, the situations are often so contrived that extrapolation to more naturalistic contexts is rendered problematic. Furthermore, there is a tendency to focus on small, isolated aspects of behavior which are more readily quantifiable, in the hope possibly that all the bits of the jigsaw will eventually fit together. The danger is that, in the lack of an appropriate overall explanatory framework, psychologists may each be working with bits of entirely different jigsaws.

Artificial intelligence

There is a wide body of work in artificial intelligence (or AI) that is concerned with natural language processing and with communication in general. Work in AI is examined that will be relevant to later discussion of the acquisition of conversational competence and the analysis of conversational disability.

What is artificial intelligence? Artificial intelligence was defined by

Minsky (1968) as "the science of making machines do things that would require intelligence if done by men". At one end of the spectrum workers in AI are attempting to produce machines that exhibit intelligent behavior – for example, expert systems that assist in mineral exploration or medical diagnosis. At the other end, research is concerned with studying the nature of intelligence through the use of computational models (Charniak and McDermott, 1985).

There are many aspects of AI that probably have little relevance to the study of pragmatic disability. However, one of the most important contributions has been the recognition of the role of world knowledge in intelligent behavior. A good example is the use of scripts to support story understanding, but there are many other aspects of knowledge representation in AI that are of potential interest to anyone involved in the study of conversational interaction (see McTear, 1987).

Scripts are a way of representing our stereotypical knowledge of the world which we rely on to make sense of stories about everyday events (Schank and Abelson, 1977). As an example, take the following short story:

Terence got on a bus to go to work. He sat down. When the conductor came, he realized that he had left his money at home, so he had to walk to work.

One way of testing a person's understanding of a story such as this is to ask the person questions about the story. Typical questions which can be answered directly from the text are:

Did Terence get on a bus to go to work?
Who came up to Terence?

However, we can also answer questions that require information not stated explicitly in the text. For example: anyone who has a basic knowledge about everyday events such as travelling on buses and getting to work would have no difficulty in answering these questions:

Did the conductor give Terence a ticket?
Was Terence late for work?

The answers to these questions might be less definite – for example, we cannot be sure that Terence was late for work, but it was likely, given that he had to walk. In other words, people are able to fill in the missing information by making inferences based on their knowledge of the situation. As with the pragmatic inferences described earlier, these inferences are not necessarily valid (as would be the case with logical inferences), but represent likely conclusions that are subject to cancellation in the light of further information.

So far there appears to be no difference between these inferences and those described in earlier sections on pragmatics, conversation analysis and psychology. Where the difference lies is not in the inferences themselves but in the explicit representation of the knowledge that makes the inferences possible. Whereas in the approaches described earlier it is simply pointed out that a person makes an inference, in AI it is necessary to specify exactly how the inference can be made so that the process can be modelled using a computer. To illustrate with the bus story example: it is suggested that people have stored in memory scripts that describe the relevant persons, objects and events occurring during a bus journey. A simple example would be the following:

Bus script

Roles	Settings
travellers	bus stop at origin of journey
bus driver	inside of bus
conductor	bus stop at destination

Props	Scenes
money for bus fare	wait for bus at bus stop
ticket exchanged for bus fare	get on bus
seat on bus	pay fare
door of bus	get off bus at destination

This script is extremely sketchy and would need to be expanded somewhat to account even for the inferences illustrated earlier. For example: the event pay fare would need to be broken down further into subevents such as produce money, issue ticket, give change. However, it can be seen even from this sketch how much knowledge is implicit when we begin to process a simple story about a bus journey. So, for example, there is no need to introduce terms such as *the conductor*, *the bus stop* or *the door*, even though they have not been previously mentioned – that is, in spite of the general rule that objects cannot be referred to using definite articles until they have first been introduced by an indefinite article. In this case it would actually be odd to say "A conductor came up to him". Furthermore, scripts provide the means to fill in information that is not made explicit in the story because it can be assumed. So, for example, even if we hear a simple story about a bus journey such as *Terence went to work by bus*, we can assume that he got on the bus at a bus stop, paid a fare, received a ticket, got off at his destination, and so on. Finally, scripts explain how we deal with unexpected events, as in our original example. As Terence did not have enough money to pay his fare, this explains why he had to walk to work. It also explains how we know that he did not receive a ticket, because events that occur in the script after offering the fare did not occur in the story as the normal course of events was interrupted at this point.

Scripts have been illustrated in some detail because they have formed the basis of some interesting research in developmental pragmatics, where investigations have been carried out into the extent of young children's world knowledge (see Chapter 6). Other important work in AI includes the study of belief systems – the difference between what different people believe about something and what they believe the other person believes about what they believe. Belief systems are the subject of much intensive research in AI, because one of the most important attributes of an intelligent and cooperative computer system would be the ability to infer its user's beliefs and needs. This ability is necessary as people do not always make explicit what they require and a helpful system would thus need to "read their mind" in order to anticipate how to provide the most helpful information. As will be seen in Chapter 6, this ability to read minds is also becoming a central focus of attention in the study of developmental pragmatics.

AI can make a useful contribution to pragmatics in two ways:

1. It requires an explicit representation of relevant background knowledge in order to support computational modelling. The benefit of this explicit representation is that the knowledge required to make inferences is clearly specified. This specification can provide a basis for the analysis of cases where background knowledge is missing or is used inappropriately – something that may underlie some of the pragmatic difficulties faced by language-impaired children.
2. It emphasizes a process-based approach, reflecting the important role of control structure in a program, but also reflecting the dynamic and changing nature of conversational contexts. Linguistics provides an explicit and rigorous account of many pragmatic phenomena, such as the nature of conversational implicature, but without specifying the actual processes involved when a person draws on background knowledge or conversational maxims to make an inference. Thus AI provides insights into process, while linguistics describes the structures involved. As a corollary, AI attends to the properties of the dialogue participants (i.e. their beliefs and mental states) while linguistics focuses on the properties of the discourse. Research in pragmatic disability also needs to focus on the mental states of the speakers in addition to analyzing what they say.

Approaches to pragmatics: some common themes

The overview of some approaches to pragmatics has indicated the diversity of issues involved in the investigation of the use of language. This diversity is partly a reflection of the disciplinary origins of each approach – for example, linguists are more concerned with how pragmatics might be justified as a level of linguistic analysis and with incorporating pragmatic analyses into existing theory; conversation analysts are interested in conversation as an example of how people interpret and manage their social activities; psychologists are concerned with understanding the processes of language comprehension and production, using the well-established techniques of experimental psychology, whereas AI workers are more concerned with the role of world knowledge in language under-standing and with devising computational models of language com-prehension and production. These interests do not necessarily coincide with those of speech–language pathologists who are more likely to be concerned with pragmatics in as much as it sheds light on the nature of speech and language disorders.

It would be useful at this point to indicate some common themes that run through these diverse approaches to the study of the use of language, especially where these common themes might be relevant to the study of pragmatic disability:

– emphasis on the functions of language rather than on its structural and formal aspects;
– analysis of larger units, such as conversations, stories, paragraphs, rather than smaller units such as sentences or words;
– attention paid to context – for example, the extralinguistic factors involved in the production and comprehension of language, rather than an analysis of decontextualized language;
– a focus on process, which involves examining the mechanisms involved in pragmatic phenomena such as making inferences;
– recognition of the role of knowledge in language production and understanding, including world (or background) knowledge as well as assumptions about the knowledge and beliefs of other people engaged in a conversation.

There are, of course, major differences in the ways in which these issues are tackled in different disciplines, as we have indicated in the overview. However, those interested in investigating pragmatic disability should be encouraged that there is sufficient common ground across different approaches to the study of the use of language to suggest that the common themes mentioned are likely to be of central significance.

Problems in applied pragmatics

This chapter is concluded with a brief look at some of the problems facing those who wish to apply pragmatics to the analysis of conversational data, with particular reference to speech–language pathologists who are interested in using concepts and insights from pragmatics to help in the identification and remediation of their clients' deficiencies in the use of language. For speech–language pathologists working in traditional areas of language analysis – phonology, syntax, lexical semantics – there is often a target norm which the patient fails to achieve, for example, because of misarticulation, an incomplete syntactic structure, or word-finding problems. Without wishing to minimize the issues involved here, it can be argued that the problems are even greater in the pragmatic domain. This point is made clearer by examining the following problem areas: identification of the unit of analysis; quantification or assessment of the extent of the problem; and making judgments concerning appropriate conversational behaviors.

Identification

Most work in applied communication (for example, social skills training) makes the assumption that communicative performance can be broken down into a set of clearly *identifiable* component skills. The speech act has been widely adopted in applied pragmatics as the basic unit of communication and studies have been concerned with the use of speech acts such as questions, requests, clarification requests. No doubt the list could also be extended to cover compliments, complaints, accusations, and many more. But how many more? Is there a finite list of such speech acts? Does the ability to use all of them (or a large subset) constitute communicative ability? Are some speech acts more important than others so that they can be prioritized in assessment and remediation?

These questions are rhetorical – no research to the authors' knowledge has attempted to confront these issues, although of course there have been various taxonomies of speech act types and some of the checklists used in the assessment of pragmatic ability (see Chapter 7) provide lists of speech acts that are used to indicate the child's level of ability in terms of number and range of speech acts used. However, in order to carry out this sort of assessment it is necessary first to identify from a conversational sample which speech acts a child is using. Given that there is no straightforward correlation between syntactic form and communicative function, as people often use indirect forms, several problems arise:

- How can we reliably identify from a particular utterance which speech act is being performed?
- How can we demonstrate that the speaker intended to convey what we have assumed to be the communicative function of the utterance and that the hearer has recognized this intention?
- How can we explain the usage of a particular indirect form – has it to do with politeness, tact, interactional pessimism?

It is not difficult to provide answers to these questions. Indeed, conversation analysts would argue that it is not possible for an analyst (or even a participant in a conversation) to determine the function of an utterance conclusively. It is important, therefore, that those wishing to investigate conversational ability (and disability) should be aware of this inherent difficulty and should be alert to the dangers of basing judgments on information that is less reliable than that provided in traditional areas of language analysis.

Quantification

Even if it were possible to identify, categorize and explain speech act usage, where would we go from here – do we count the number of times a person asks questions or pays compliments (appropriately)? Is the number of occurrences of a speech act significant as a measure of communicative ability or is it perhaps the range of speech acts used?

Related to this point is the problem that the focus on speech acts has wrongly placed an emphasis on isolated behaviors, whereas here the concern is with communication – that is, an interpersonal behavior. Thus, as mentioned earlier in relation to the emphasis of conversation analysis on conversation as an interactional and collaborative achievement, the use of a particular speech act has to be seen not only in relation to a speaker's overall communicative aims (for example, to achieve the goal of wheedling a favor from someone), but in relation to the other person's behaviors. As Levinson (1983, p.294) has written:

> Conversation is not a structured product in the same way that a sentence is – it is rather the outcome of the interaction of two or more independent, goal-directed individuals, with often divergent interests.

Looking at the practical consequences of this, it is necessary to consider to what extent a person's use of particular speech acts is *dependent on* the other person's behaviors. Thus it is senseless to count the number of times a person asks questions in an interaction without considering how the other person's behaviors may have constrained or encouraged questioning in the first place. What is important is the interaction between the two conversational partners, because the behavior of one participant cannot be understood without reference to the behavior of the other participant. This important issue is dealt with again in Chapter 3.

Of course it could be argued that there are practical advantages in working with checklists of target behaviors that we can observe, quantify, and, on the basis of such analysis, incorporate in programs of intervention. The use of checklists of pragmatic behavior is examined in greater detail in Chapter 7. For the moment it is agreed that in practice clinicians and researchers have been able to isolate particular deficiencies in some aspect of language use and to devise programs of intervention that may have brought about acceptable improvements. However, it is important to avoid the danger of confining attention to those aspects of communication that are more easily identified and quantified, or, even worse, the danger of coming to believe that this is all that communication is about.

Appropriacy

Appropriacy is a central concern of pragmatics. Indeed, as shown in Chapter 1, one definition of pragmatics is in terms of the study of the appropriate use of language – for example, knowing when to use a more polite request because you are talking to someone of higher status or because you are asking a favor, or knowing how to make an appropriate response to what someone else has just said. Many studies of children's pragmatic ability include categories such as "appropriate content" to cater for just this aspect of language behavior.

Appropriacy would also appear to have empirical support as a discriminating factor in comparisons of different types of language-disabled children. For example, in a recent study it was found that children, who had been categorized on independent grounds as having semantic –pragmatic disability, were primarily deficient in terms of the appropriacy of their use of language, as compared to other children with more traditional language deficits (Bishop and Adams, 1989).

What then are the problems with appropriacy? One problem is that appropriacy (or more accurately judgments of appropriacy) is relative, rather than categorical. Thus, whereas it is generally easier to make judgments of well-formedness in phonology and syntax, in pragmatics it is more *a matter of degree*. To take a simple example: an utterance might be judged to be reasonably appropriate in terms of politeness but still either more polite than required or perhaps less polite than required. However, the judgments are being made from the point of view of an outside observer (or analyst), whereas the participants themselves may have found the utterance to be perfectly appropriate. In any case, it will not fail in its communicative function but may convey some additional information if its recipient does indeed perceive it to be either too polite or not polite enough.

Furthermore, as the appropriacy of an utterance depends on a variety of linguistic and extralinguistic factors, such as the relative status of speaker and hearer, what has previously been discussed, the current physical context, and the goals of the participants, there are many different ways in which an utterance might be inappropriate on one dimension but appropriate on others. In other words, appropriacy is not a unitary phenomenon.

However, the most problematic issue for the notion of appropriacy is what Grice has termed "exploitation" – that is, the ability of speakers to exploit the conventional use of language to convey some additional message. Thus instead of appearing to be inappropriate, a person might be acting inventively. The typical examples are irony and humour, but such exploitation of normal conventions is pervasive in human communication and it is in fact the inability to make the necessary inferences that will make sense of such cases that is a characteristic feature of some children suffering from pragmatic disability. So, although in practice researchers provide the safeguard of conducting inter-observer reliability tests when making judgments of appropriacy, there is still the danger of labelling an utterance as inappropriate when in fact the speaker has tried, perhaps unsuccessfully, to convey some additional meaning through exploitation. A simple example would be when a child's utterance is labelled as inappropriate whereas perhaps the child was trying to be humorous. In this case, we might be dealing with an inability to carry off a joke (which itself is a pragmatic phenomenon) rather than an inability to respond appropriately to another's talk.

In other words, appropriacy does not appear to be so much rule-based as *principle-based*, and there is always the issue of defeasibility (i.e. that the inference can be cancelled). Furthermore, successful communication is a cooperatively and interactionally achieved accomplishment involving complex interpretative skills and the utilization of a wide range of background knowledge. What this means is that it is not possible in principle to observe an interaction and make judgments of appropriacy. Rather what is appropriate is what the participants themselves accept as appropriate in the interaction.

Concluding remarks

In this chapter a review was made of those aspects of research in pragmatics and the study of language use that are particularly relevant for speech–language pathologists interested in investigating pragmatic disability. One of the aims has been to persuade readers that it is important to adopt a coherent and consistent theoretical framework rather than borrowing bits and pieces from a variety of frameworks which are possibly incompatible. At the same time hopefully pathologists have been encouraged to develop a healthy skepticism towards attempts to put ideas too quickly into practice before they are fully understood.

Thus, as suggested, there are several difficulties when applying pragmatic concepts to the analysis of conversational data. This does not mean, of course, that we should throw up our hands in despair and stick to those aspects of language that are more manageable. The problems that children have in using language are real enough. It is necessary to develop ways of understanding these problems and methods for helping the children to overcome them. It is the authors' belief that much is to be learned from theoretical and empirical studies of conversation. Speech–language pathologists can contribute to our greater understanding of these issues through their own observations and analyses of the children they encounter with pragmatic disability.

In brief, some of the problems that confront those wishing to apply pragmatics to speech–language pathology are:

– The diversity of approaches to pragmatic phenomena.
– The problem of translating theory into practice – for example, finding aspects of communicative ability that can be observed and assessed, and then devising suitable programs of intervention.

Bearing these problems in mind, the question of pragmatic disability in children can now be looked at. In the next chapter ways of studying pragmatic development in children are reviewed; it is shown in particular how the choice of a particular method has a crucial bearing on the sorts of results obtained. It will be important to bear this factor in mind when findings from studies of pragmatic development and pragmatic disability are reviewed in subsequent chapters.

Chapter 3
Studying Pragmatic Disability

The term "pragmatic disability" has been used to refer to problems that children experience in using language to communicate. These problems are sufficiently severe to have a profound effect on children's ability to perform adequately at school. They may also make it more difficult for the children to make friends and cope satisfactorily in everyday social contexts. Yet the nature of the problems is not always obvious, nor is there necessarily any satisfactory explanation. For those concerned professionally with language- and communication-impaired children, such as speech–language pathologists and teachers, it is important to have an understanding of pragmatic disability, what forms it takes, how it relates to other abilities – both linguistic and nonlinguistic – and how it might be assessed and treated.

In this chapter the concern is with how pragmatic disability has been studied and with the implications of adopting a particular research strategy for our understanding of the nature and explanation of pragmatic disability. In subsequent chapters the nature of pragmatic disability is examined and its relationship to children's linguistic and other abilities addressed. However, at the start it will be useful to examine some terminology that is commonly used in the field of pragmatic disability.

Terminology

The term "pragmatic disability" is being used as a fairly neutral way of referring to children's difficulties in using language. Various other terms are in common use, such as semantic–pragmatic disorder, fluent language disorder, and atypical pervasive developmental disorder, and investigations of the nature of these dysfunctions have given rise to attempts to redefine and explain clinical classifications such as infantile autism and Asperger's syndrome. Bishop (1989) provides a clear discussion of these categories and of the boundaries between them.

It will be helpful to examine more closely the term "semantic–pragmatic disorder" (SPD), because it is widely used and yet is rather unsatisfactory in several ways. This term is derived from a classification of subtypes of developmental language disorders by Rapin and Allen (1987). Rapin and Allen distinguished between several subtypes of developmental language disorder, including phonologic–syntactic syndrome and semantic–pragmatic syndrome. Children with phonologic–syntactic syndrome were characterized by difficulties with language form, in particular, with phonological or syntactic aspects of language (or both). They did not have problems with using language for communication. In comparison, a different group of children had relatively little difficulty with language form, but had difficulty in using and understanding language in communicative situations. The term "semantic–pragmatic syndrome" was coined to refer to this group of children.

There are some problems with this terminology. On the one hand, the use of the description "semantic–pragmatic" is intended to encompass aspects of meaning and language use. However, pairing together "semantic" and "pragmatic" obscures the differences between these levels of language. As explained in Chapters 1 and 2, semantics should be used to refer to those aspects of meaning that are conventional and part of a language system. Pragmatics refers to those aspects of meaning that are nonconventional, for example, inferences based on principles of communication such as Gricean maxims. At the pragmatic level it is possible for an utterance to mean more than it says in a literal sense. More generally, pragmatics is used to refer to principles that govern the use of language in context, including the structure of conversation. Putting together the terms "semantic" and "pragmatic" only obscures these issues and may prevent us from locating and explaining the nature of the child's difficulties.

A further problem is that the proposed distinction between children with difficulties in language form and those with difficulties in language use suggests that formal and communicative aspects of language are unrelated. It also suggests that language disabilities fall neatly into these groupings. So, for example, it might be assumed that children with pragmatic difficulties have no problems in producing grammatically well-formed sentences. The evidence does not support this view, as will be seen later. Furthermore, there could be a more indirect link between grammatical difficulties and pragmatic disability, because there is evidence that some children with pragmatic difficulties had a previous history of language impairment of a grammatical nature.

In this book the more neutral term "pragmatic disability" will be used, though this term still creates problems because it implies an identifiable disability. An alternative possibility is that what are observed are difficulties with the use of language which can be described using concepts from pragmatics but which have their origins in some other clinically identifiable disability. Discussion of these issues will be postponed until after the relevant background has been discussed in later chapters.

Investigating children's pragmatic development: experimental and naturalistic methods

The study of children's communicative development has followed two distinct paths (Dickson, 1982). Experimental studies, based on artificial tasks performed in laboratory settings and referred to widely as studies of *referential communication*, have tended to support the view that children's early communication is deficient (Flavell et al.,, 1968; Krauss and Glucksberg, 1969). However, observational studies conducted under more naturalistic conditions have tended to support the view that even very young children demonstrate a high degree of communicative proficiency (Maratsos, 1973; Shatz and Gelman, 1973; McTear, 1985a). It will be important to consider these different sets of findings for two reasons: first it is necessary to explain why they have reached such seemingly incompatible conclusions and, secondly, because both methods are used for the assessment of children with pragmatic disability, it is necessary to appreciate the reliability and usefulness of each approach.

Studies of referential communication are concerned mainly with relating communicative ability to aspects of cognitive development such as childhood egocentrism. Egocentrism is a theoretical construct, first proposed by Piaget (1926), to explain children's communicative deficiencies. Briefly, egocentrism refers to a failure to address or adapt information to the needs of a listener. Experiments designed to test the theory of childhood egocentrism have typically involved tasks in which a speaker and listener are separated by a screen (in order to prevent nonverbal communication) and the speaker has to communicate some information to the listener. Although the task is artificial, it permits some control over the situation which is not possible in more naturalistic settings, thus giving referential communication tasks some degree of face validity.

The concern with egocentrism has tended to obscure the fact that two different types of skill are involved in experimental studies of referential communication (Shantz, 1981):

- the ability to describe objects accurately so that they can be distinguished from other objects;
- the ability to take the listener's perspective and to adapt the information to the needs of the listener.

The first set of skills involves making descriptions and comparisons and depends on the ability to decide what the distinguishing attributes of an object are as well as on the linguistic ability to encode these distinctions. Typically the child playing the role of the speaker is required to describe certain objects or shapes from an array so that the listener, who has a similar array, can select the correct items. It is clear that these skills are concerned with the informational adequacy of a message and need not involve an assessment of the listener's perspective.

The second set of skills is concerned with whether the child can adapt the message to the needs of the listener and involve what has been referred to as *role-taking ability*. One commonly used technique is to use different types of listener. For example, listeners might be blindfolded or might have different amounts of knowledge. In the first case the child has to deliver a message that is comprehensible to a listener who cannot see the objects being described, while in the second it is necessary to adapt the description to take account of what the listener knows and does not know.

Studies of referential communication have been criticized on several grounds. One problem is their artificiality, as already mentioned. A second problem is that many of the tasks used in the experiments were too abstract and difficult for the children so that failure could be attributed to other factors, such as a lack of appropriate vocabulary to describe the criterial features of an object, rather than to a lack of role-taking ability. When more child-oriented tasks were used and children were adequately instructed in the requirements of the task, they often demonstrated role-taking abilities in advance of the predictions of Piaget's theory of egocentrism (Donaldson, 1978). Furthermore, results from these studies often conflicted with observations of children's ability to adapt their talk to their listeners, particularly when they were required to simplify their message to suit the needs of younger listeners (Shatz and Gelman, 1973). Finally, because these studies focus on communication solely in terms of the transmission of information, they overlook other aspects of communicative ability such as turn-taking, responding to the previous speaker's utterance, or making inferences about what the other speaker intended to convey.

Naturalistic studies of communicative development have tended to examine the social context of communication, such as the nature of interaction between children and different types of conversational partner, as well as the ability of children to participate in different types of speech events. These studies have emphasized the competence of young children, in contrast to the experimental studies. Some aspects of naturalistic studies are described in the next sections. However, it should also be pointed out that naturalistic studies have certain disadvantages. Because the situations are natural and spontaneous, the observer has little control over the data and has to work with whatever data happen to emerge. This results in problems of quantifying the data in any reliable way and of making any useful comparisons across samples. However, naturalistic studies have provided a rich source of information about young children's communicative development as well as providing useful hypotheses that can be further tested under more controlled conditions. In subsequent chapters several different aspects of communicative development will be reviewed, drawing on experimental and observational studies where relevant, because both approaches provide complementary perspectives and methodologies.

How is pragmatic disability studied?

There are three main ways in which researchers have tried to investigate pragmatic disability: (1) group design studies; (2) case studies; (3) group comparisons. Each of these methods has advantages and disadvantages. However, it is important to realize that the choice of a particular method can determine the sorts of questions that are available for investigation. For this reason not only will the methods be examined but also an indication given of how they may or may not be useful as ways of reaching a better understanding of pragmatic disability.

Group design studies

Group design studies are based on the assumption that children can be assigned to discrete groups which can then be compared or subjected to some experimental condition. The advantage of group design studies is that they should provide more general indicators than case studies, which may be dealing with idiosyncratic and atypical cases.

As far as research in pragmatic disability is concerned, the approach used in group design studies is to examine language-impaired children in comparison with language-matched and age-matched peers. Part of the motivation for these studies is the attempt to extend linguistic analysis beyond the more traditional levels of phonology, syntax, and semantics, to focus on context, discourse, and pragmatics. There is also the attempt to explore the possibility of whether language-impaired children have problems at the pragmatic level.

The general design of these studies is that a group of language-impaired children is compared on selected pragmatic skills with a group of age-matched and a group of language-matched peers (Figure 3.1).For example, a pragmatic skill, such as the use of clarification requests to resolve misunderstandings, is selected and the different groups are examined for their use of this skill. The usual prediction is that the language-impaired children will be inferior to their age-matched peers, because it is assumed that their use of language is closely related to their level of linguistic development – more specifically, that their deficiencies in language structure will affect their ability to use language. Consequently it will also be predicted that their performance will be similar to that of their language–matched peers.

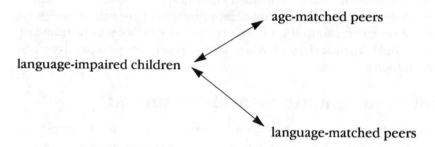

Figure 3.1 Comparisons made in group design studies

Findings from group design studies
Results from group design studies have tended to both support and disconfirm these predictions, or to support them for some pragmatic variables but not for others (for comprehensive reviews, see Fey and Leonard, 1983; Bryan, 1986; Donahue, 1987; see also Chapter 5).

In order to explain these discrepant findings, it is necessary to examine the main assumption on which group design studies of pragmatic disability are based – that language impairment predicts pragmatic disability. The relationship between pragmatic ability and language development will be examined in greater detail in Chapter 5. For the moment, however, it can be noted that, although the hypothesis that language impairment predicts pragmatic disability has been upheld in many studies, several other studies have failed to support this hypothesis, or, more subtly, that they have supported it for some pragmatic variables but not for others. What this suggests is that a more fine-grained approach is required to the study of pragmatic disability.

Group design studies depend crucially on appropriate measures for matching groups – in particular, for level of language. In many cases the criteria used to select and match groups are often imprecise or too global. Measures such as the mean length of utterance (MLU) are often used. However, MLU is a rather global measure which becomes less reliable as a way of grouping children as their language develops beyond the early stages, and in any case it is not always clear whether MLU can be correlated clearly with structural stages (Crystal, 1974; Miller, 1981; Klee and Fitzgerald, 1985; Klee et al., 1989). Furthermore, grouping together a number of language-impaired children assumes that they constitute a homogeneous group. Unless the linguistic measures on which these groupings are made are precise, it is likely that many different levels and types of disability will be subsumed under the one label. Some investigators have made some progress along these lines by using various measures of expressive and receptive language ability as well as tests of cognitive development that have led to more precise statements of possible relationships between language ability and pragmatic skills (Leonard, 1986; Hargrove, Straka and Medders, 1988; Craig and Evans, 1989).

Even if there are more accurate criteria for matching groups of subjects, there is a further problem of explaining how specific structural deficiencies give rise to pragmatic disability. To take an example: if a child is classified as being language-impaired on the basis of grammatical immaturity, what effect might this impairment have on the ability to make clarification requests? If it could be shown that there was a close correspondence between the grammatical structures in which the child was deficient and those needed to make clarification requests, then we might be confident in assuming some relationship between language impairment and pragmatic disability. However, it is possible for a child to know the syntactic structures that are necessary for accomplishing a particular communicative function, and to use these structures for other purposes, but to still remain deficient in respect of the communicative function in question. In other words, the use of a particular pragmatic skill might be related to factors that have nothing to do with a child's formal linguistic abilities. These factors need to be considered fully before assumptions are made about unidirectional relationships between language impairment and pragmatic disability.

Measuring pragmatic ability also poses problems because there is not always a straightforward linear relationship between development and the extent to which a child performs a particular communicative function. A child may produce more polite requests but it is also necessary to examine whether these are being used appropriately (Donahue, 1981). Similarly, we would expect a decrease in certain behaviors, such as conversational dysfluencies or overlapped turns. However, we need to consider carefully the nature of the behaviors and the circumstances under which they are produced. Conversational dysfluencies could be evidence that the child is experiencing difficulties, as MacLachlan and Chapman (1988) propose as an explanation of their finding that language-impaired children produced more dysfluencies than other groups in a narrative task. However, an increase in conversational dysfluencies can indicate that the child's self-monitoring skills have improved (Evans, 1985). Similarly, while turn-internal overlaps may indicate that the child is unable to process the ongoing turn in order to interrupt at appropriate places in the utterance, an increase in overlapped turns may be evidence of a more sophisticated turn-taking ability in which the child attempts to predict the potential point at which the current turn is complete (Craig and Evans, 1989). Thus we need to examine pragmatic behaviors both qualitatively and quantitatively before attempting to explain the development of these behaviors in terms of linguistic and other abilities.

Finally, it is possible that there are different types of pragmatic disability, some of which may be either directly or indirectly related to language impairment, and others which may be almost totally unrelated. If this is the case, then it is no wonder that the major predictions of group design studies have sometimes been disconfirmed and that the general picture is one of confusion. An attempt will be made to resolve this confusion in Chapters 5 and 6 in which different types of pragmatic disability are discussed in detail .

To summarize, group design studies have provided information on questions concerning the relationship between linguistic impairment and pragmatic disability. However, the contradictory results indicate some of the methodological problems in this area and the need for more sophisticated approaches. The main problems with group design studies are as follows:

- There is a lack of precision in the criteria used for selection of groups.
- There is an assumption that language-impaired children constitute a homogeneous group.
- There is a restriction on investigations of pragmatic disability to children who are defined as language-impaired in the first place, so that other children with pragmatic difficulties but without language impairment may be overlooked.
- Pragmatic behaviors are often analysed superficially without regard to the context in which they were produced.
- There is a tendency towards post-hoc explanations of possible corre-lations between language impairment and pragmatic disability, based on whatever findings emerge from particular studies rather than on a theory-driven model of these relationships.
- There is little or no attempt to consider relationships between specific linguistic skills, specific social and cognitive skills, and specific pragmatic behaviors.

Some of these problems are addressed in case studies and group comparison studies, which will be described in the next two sections.

Case studies of pragmatic disability

Case studies provide a means of investigating in depth children who have been identified as having a pragmatic disability. Early case studies were interesting as they suggested the possibility that some children might be impaired only in their pragmatic skills – in other words, that pragmatic disability could exist independently of or in the absence of other impairments (Bloom and Lahey, 1978). In this section the results of some case studies are summarized and then a critical evaluation made of the usefulness of case studies as a method for investigating pragmatic disability.

A case study by Blank, Gessner and Esposito (1979) was the first case study to describe pragmatic disability (although the authors did not use this term in their paper). Blank, Gessner and Esposito described a 3-year-old boy whose language was syntactically and semantically well developed but who lacked the ability to communicate. The child's utterances were well-formed in respect of his age but were deficient as conversational contributions. In particular this child often failed to respond or produced inappropriate responses. The following is a typical example (Blank, Gessner and Esposito, 1979, p. 346):

(Father and child are looking at a book)

Father	John
That's Pat's house. What's everyone doing at Pat's house?	
	knock, knock, knock (knocking on door in book)
Come in	
	Nobody's home
Nobody's home? Well, isn't Pat home? (Pat is evident in the picture)	
	Come back later
OK, let's go to Pat's new house	
	Pat's old house

In this example John's father tries to initiate conversation by asking questions and he also tries to sustain the conversation by responding to John's utterances despite their apparent lack of relevance. John's contributions follow the sort of routine that he may have heard from his parents when they called on someone who was not at home. However, this routine is inappropriate here because in the picture provided with the script it is evident that Pat is at home. John appears unable to adapt his routine to the current context. This mode of behavior makes communication difficult and places the main responsibility for conversational success on the father who tries to make John's utterances appear relevant. Indeed, as Blank and co-workers point out, any successful conversational exchanges that occurred could be attributed to the parents' responsiveness to whatever John happened to say rather than to any skill on John's part in initiating or sustaining the conversation.

A similar case of pragmatic disability in the absence of other linguistic impairments is found in Greenlee's (1981) case study which was referred to briefly in Chapter 1. The child in this study (Rodney) – an 8-year-old boy diagnosed with an organic brain disorder (tuberous sclerosis) and childhood psychosis – was characterized by deviant patterns in his use of language, although he was similar in respect of his expressive and receptive language abilities to children of a comparable mental age. Some of the features that Greenlee identified as unusual were:

– The use of *what's that – an X* sequences (e.g. "What's that – a chair"), in which the child both asked and answered the question. Although such sequences are sometimes produced by very young children aged 2 or 3 years, they are most unusual in children of this age and at this stage of language development.
– Combinations of portions of his conversational partners' utterances in his own utterances – for example:
    Adult: Let's see, what shall we draw?
    Rodney: Shall we draw, so you could take it home?

Here the child combines part of the adult's utterance into his own utterance. A similar strategy has been reported in the language of autistic children (Baltaxe and Simmons, 1977). The result is often an agrammatical or meaningless sentence.

– Problems in pronoun reference – for example, the use of both first and second person pronouns to refer to himself, or, as in this example, the use of third person reference:
    (Rodney and adult are in the playroom just after lunch)
    Rodney: C'mere, c'mere. He don't eat no ice cream
    Adult: (approaches Rodney) Who?
    Rodney: Rodney don't eat no ice cream
    Adult: Why?
    Rodney: Rodney don't eat no ice cream. You don't eat no ice cream 'til tomorrow

As a result of the regular use of these features, it was difficult to make sense of much of Rodney's talk, especially as attempts to clarify were either responded to inappropriately or not at all.

In summary, as Greenlee points out, this child presents a cluster of features that occur rarely or only at very early stages in normally developing children. It is this combination of unusual features, together with his inability to repair conversational breakdowns, which accounts for the child's deviant patterns of language use.

One further case study that can be mentioned is of a 10-year-old boy in full day-time attendance at a special language unit (McTear, 1985b). Although this child had no obvious difficulties with syntactic structures, his conversation had been described by speech–language pathologists and teachers as "bizarre and confused" and as "stilted and formal". The case study was an attempt to describe these features in some detail.

The main points to note in this case study concerned the nature of the child's responses in conversation and the informational content of his contributions. As far as responses were concerned, two aspects were noteworthy. First, it was found that the child tended to produce minimal responses but failed to provide any additional material, so that much of the conversational initiative was left to his conversational partner. This may be partly attributable to the fact that the data obtained were from conversations with adults, in which the relationships were asymmetrical. However, as his speech–language pathologist and teachers reported, he also engaged in little interaction with his peers and seemed happier to interact with adults. Thus, although he lacked assertiveness, he seemed to enjoy participating in conversations with adults and was perhaps constrained by an inability to process language sufficiently to enable him to adopt a more assertive role.

The second characteristic of this child's responses was that, although he rarely added new content, he failed to use ellipsis appropriately, with the result that his utterances often appeared repetitive and redundant. For example:

Adult: Are they friends of yours?
Child: They are friends of mine

However, the most striking aspect of conversations with the child concerned the content of his contributions. It was often difficult to assess the factual accuracy of his utterances and to discern causal and sequential relations in his descriptions of events such as his daily journey from home to school. An example was presented in Chapter 1 where he showed confusion concerning a forthcoming sports day at his school. In some cases simple misunderstandings may have been the source of the difficulty. However, a cumulation of misunderstandings and contradictions, including confusions about the membership of his family, his journey to school and out-of-school activities, suggests a deficiency in his ability to handle information, particularly his ability to describe sequences of events and to understand how events are related temporally and causally. Some further examples from this child will be presented in Chapter 6 and the nature of his pragmatic disability explored further.

At this point it is necessary to pause and evaluate the strengths and weaknesses of case studies such as these. One obvious advantage is that case studies provide a description of children with pragmatic disability without language impairment who might otherwise have escaped attention in traditional group design studies. Case studies also result in more in-depth analysis than is possible in comparative studies. In McTear's study, for example, a detailed sequential analysis of conversations with the child, as opposed to a quantification of selected items such as number and range of speech acts used or length and nature of inter-turn pauses, provided empirical support for the general impressions of "bizarre and confused" conversations which had been reported of this child. A further advantage of case studies is that, by treating the child as unique and identifying each individual child's specific problems, it is possible to plan more individualized programs of remediation.

However, there is a danger in proliferating case studies in the absence of a satisfactory descriptive and explanatory framework. Early case studies fulfilled a need in that they identified and described discourse and conversational problems experienced by some children. Without some basis for comparison across case studies, however, there is no opportunity to generalize from individual cases to more general principles. Moreover, in the absence of more detailed information about the child, it is not possible to explore potential relationships between the child's conversational deficiencies and any linguistic or nonlinguistic problems. Without such information no serious explanations for the child's problems can be offered. McTear (1985b) explained some of the problems of the child in his case study in terms of deficient world knowledge, but in general case studies tend to simply report the most striking features and run the risk of tending towards the anecdotal. Finally, case studies provide a snapshot of a child at a particular point in time and thus do not offer information about developmental patterns or previous history of difficulties.

One case study that overcame some of these problems was a longitudinal study by Conti-Ramsden and Gunn (1986). These researchers observed a 3-year-old boy named Tony for a period of $3\frac{1}{2}$ years in an attempt to document changes in the child's profile across time. In the area of pragmatic development, Tony began to respond in conversation well before he began to initiate conversations spontaneously. In addition, Tony began using language spontaneously mainly to label and describe and it was only when he was nearing 6 years of age that he used language to request information and/or action. Such late emergence of requests in the presence of enough expressive language to enable their formulation represents a deviant pattern of development which affected the quality and quantity of Tony's social interaction with peers and adults. The question then arises as to why this may be the case. Conti-Ramsden and Gunn also looked at other related areas of development in order to explore potential relationships between conversational problems and other nonlinguistic or linguistic difficulties.

In the area of verbal comprehension, Tony's profile was uneven across and within time. At any particular point, Tony could achieve later milestones, e.g. choose an object by shape and colour, while unable to succeed in simple interactional acts, e.g. look attentively or smile appropriately. As Tony grew older he became better at scoring in standardized tests and the tests thus became worse at pinpointing Tony's difficulties with verbal reasoning and inferencing (answering Wh-questions, especially *why*) and interpersonal understanding (taking the other person's perspective, e.g. How do they feel? What do they need to know in order to understand?). In terms of nonverbal abilities, Tony's profile was totally uneventful and he consistently scored above his age level in nonverbal tests of intelligence. The authors argue that this is not to suggest that Tony was cognitively intact, but that such tests are too global and fail to capture specific cognitive difficulties, especially those that may underlie verbal–pragmatic problems. In the same vein, Conti-Ramsden and Gunn argue that the typical picture of good expressive language (syntax and phonology) in children with pragmatic disabilities, although true in relative terms, was not so in more complex and subtle ways. For example, they found Tony had difficulties in marking tense appropriately in discourse (dialogue and narrative).

The study of Conti-Ramsden and Gunn (1986) therefore advanced our knowledge in principle but fell short of providing answers in practice. The tools currently available to tap children's linguistic and nonlinguistic difficulties are blunt when it comes to applying them to pragmatic difficulties and we need to think again. This state of affairs is related to the absence of a satisfactory descriptive and explanatory framework. As such a framework evolves, so will the means for investigation.

To summarize the main strengths of case studies:

- They permit an in-depth study of a particular child.
- They permit the particular characteristics of a child, such as unusual use of language, to be investigated without preconceptions about the influence of other factors such as the child's linguistic, cognitive or social development.
- In a longitudinal study, they can show how a child's use of language develops (or fails to develop) over time.

It is also important to consider some of the disadvantages of case studies:

- There may be difficulty in making comparisons across different case studies unless consistent descriptive frameworks are used.
- Unless there is sufficient detail on a range of aspects related to the

child's language use – such as the child's linguistic, cognitive, social and emotional development – then it will not be possible to explain the child's difficulties in the use of language.
– Unless a longitudinal study is conducted, we will only see a snapshot of a child's performance at a particular point in time and will not be able to make connections with earlier or later developments.

Group comparison studies

In the previous sections it was shown how group design studies are often based on invalid assumptions about the relationship between language impairment and pragmatic disability, while case studies suffer from a lack of generality. A third approach – large-scale group comparison studies – seems to offer a promising way forward. These studies involve the use of pragmatic protocols that are used to classify a range of pragmatic behaviors across a sample of children (and adults) exhibiting different language disabilities. It will be helpful to illustrate these points with two examples of group comparison studies.

The work of Prutting and Kirchner (1987) is based on the assumption that a global appraisal of a child's or adult's communicative system can provide important information. With this in mind, they developed an observational protocol that was simple to use and yielded high levels of inter-observer reliability. The pragmatic protocol involved judgments of appropriateness and inappropriateness for a wide range of pragmatic behaviors. These behaviors were separated into three major categories: verbal aspects, paralinguistic aspects, and nonverbal aspects. In the verbal area, judgments are made with respect to speech acts, topic selection, turn-taking, and cohesion among others. Paralinguistic factors included intelligibility, prosody, fluency, and vocal characteristics. Finally, nonverbal elements addressed issues such as physical proximity, body posture, gestures, facial expression, and eye gaze.

Prutting and Kirchner (1987) applied the pragmatic protocol to 157 subjects during a 15-minute conversation with a familiar partner. The judgments were made on-line while observing the interaction. The subjects included 42 children with language disorders, 42 children with articulation disorders, 42 children developing language normally, 11 adults following a left hemisphere cerebrovascular accident, 10 adults following a right hemisphere cerebrovascular accident, and 10 adults with normal language. Interestingly, these researchers found that the pragmatic protocol was able to produce profiles that identified and separated the four distinct clinical groups from each other as well as from normal children and adults. Nonetheless, the data which formed the basis for differentiating the groups were few in absolute terms, that is, the mean percentage of inappropriate pragmatic parameters for the children with articulation disorders was only 4 percent, for the language-disordered group it was 12 percent, for adults with left hemisphere lesions it was 18 percent, and for adults with right hemisphere lesions it was 14 percent. In addition, there was a great deal of variability within each group. This variability, they acknowledge, probably represents the existence of subgroups within these large clinical categories such as language disorders which points to the need for further work on individual differences. Thus, an observational schedule such as the pragmatic protocol that involves simple judgments of appropriacy can be useful as a general communicative index but cannot provide information as to why certain behaviors are inappropriate or in what way they are inappropriate, or how they may related to other appropriate or inappropriate behaviors.

In this vein, the work of Bishop and Adams (1989) and Adams and Bishop (1989) goes several steps further. These researchers investigated conversational characteristics of children with pragmatic disability from two perspectives. One perspective involved, much like Prutting and Kirchner (1987), the examination of natural conversations of different groups of language-disordered children in an attempt to identify specific behaviors that differentiated clinical groups. The second approach involved identifying episodes of inappropriate conversational behaviors and attempting to categorize them in order to gain some insight as to the nature of the children's difficulties. Bishop and Adams used an audio-taped, semi-structured situation involving looking at photographs to obtain 5–10 minutes' conversational interactions between children and a female adult stranger. The conversation was allowed to develop naturally but the adult could refer to a set of prepared questions when necessary. A sample of 57 language-impaired children participated in the study which could be broadly divided into two groups. Fourteen children appeared to fall within the category of pragmatic disorders and 43 children fell within the category of other language disorders. In addition, approximately 60 normal control children ranging in age from 4 to 12 years were included.

Bishop and Adams (1989) included in their conversational analysis an examination of exchange structure, turn-taking, repairs and cohesion. Their analysis went further than Prutting and Kirchner's (1987) in that it did not simply make judgments as to whether a pragmatic deficit was absent or present, but involved characterizing the conversation, and transcribing and coding each conversational turn. Using this procedure, they found that children with pragmatic disability produced more initiations than other language-disordered children and this appeared to be the one area that differentiated the groups. Exchange structure, repairs and cohesion were not found to yield differences. In the same vein, they found that adults exhibited difficulties in conversing with pragmatically disordered children. Adults had a higher frequency of interrupts and requests for clarification when interacting with the aforementioned children. Nonetheless, Bishop and Adams also found that their more refined coding scheme was not always reliable. Conversational behaviors falling within the categories of turn-taking and repair yielded low levels of inter-rater reliability which brings to the forefront the important question of what the criteria are for making decisions about children's and adult's conversational behaviors. This question is particularly relevant when Adams and Bishop (1989) attempt their second approach and categorize inappropriate conversational behaviors in different categories, not all of which yielded reliable results. There appears to be a great need for further research on developing and refining data-driven categories which make sense within theory but are reliable in practice. Adams and Bishop also point to the important fact that some of their categories appear to be closely linked to cognitive abilities rather than to linguistic ones which raises the question of the consistency or lack thereof of analytical systems used to examine conversational ability. Research to develop consistent criteria for describing and explaining inappropriate conversational behavior is sorely needed. Nevertheless, the work of Bishop and Adams (1989) and Adams and Bishop (1989) combined represents an important step forward in that a group comparison study is complemented by an in-depth look at problematic episodes which are then further examined. This particular combination allows for generalizability without necessarily sacrificing individual differences.

A summary of the strengths of large-scale group comparison studies is as follows:

- They are sufficiently large scale to permit the derivation of more general findings compared with case studies.
- They avoid the problem of overly delimiting the issues to be investigated which characterizes group-design studies comparing language-impaired with normally developing children.
- They permit constellations of disabilities to emerge and the correlation of these constellations with groups of children classified in terms of medical or linguistic categories.

However, there are also some problems with group comparison studies:

- They are only as adequate as the theory of pragmatic competence that underlies them.
- They tend to restrict the data (for the sake of manageability) to a sample of 10–20 minutes' conversation, which may be spontaneous (and so less amenable to comparative analysis) or more structured (and so less naturalistic).

The need for an interactional framework

The notion that human beings engage in social interaction has been at the basis of much recent work in parent–child and clinician–client interaction, yet by and large the methods so far described have failed to consider sufficiently the interactional aspects of children's language use. One visible contribution of pragmatics to the work of speech–language pathologists is that it has promoted a greater emphasis on the contextual aspects of communication and, in particular, on the interactional contexts in which children learn and use language. It is now time to analyze the interactional context of language development and use in more detail. To start with a framework is provided for the study of parent–child interaction. This framework is used to examine the nature of clinician–child discourse when discussing issues of intervention in Chapter 8.

The interactional framework

As suggested previously, a broad view of pragmatics encompasses much more than just another set of linguistic skills. It provides an integrative view of the child's development where the child is inextricably linked to the social environment and the social environment has a direct effect on the child. Thus, in order to understand how the child develops communicative competence, it is necessary to know in what contexts and under what conditions the child uses and learns language. Corsaro (1981) points to the well-known fact that language is acquired and used in social contexts. Furthermore, the aim of learning language is to be able to share communicative functions with others. Developmentally, children are linked to significant people with whom they interact and learn. Figure 3.2 below presents the developmental progression of significant others in the child's life based on the work of Corsaro (1981).

1. CAREGIVER(S)–INFANT

2. CAREGIVER-MEDIATED INTERACTION

    (a) CHILD——-ADULT

        caregiver

    (b) CHILD——-CHILD

        caregiver

3. CHILD – CHILD PEER INTERACTION

4. ADULT – CHILD INTERACTION

5. ADULT – ADULT

Figure 3.2 Social contexts in the child's development

Early in the child's life, the caregiver and child are a closely knit dyad. As will be discussed later, parent–child interactions and routines form the basis from which children's early language develops. As children grow older, caregivers continue to be the major agents of the child's social-ization as they continue to interact with the child and act as mediators between the child and other adults and children. Consequently, the contexts within which the child can interact grow to include adult–child-mediated interactions and child–child-mediated interactions. As time passes and children begin to attend playgroups, nurseries, or other pre-school provisions, the child is more frequently engaged in peer interactions. This context is of particular importance as the situation of children interacting with other children provides experience where the two interactants are of the same status; thus this alignment extends the horizons of the young language-learning child significantly. At this time, other adults enter the social scene of the child such as teachers, and for some children, clinicians. Finally, as children grow into young adults peer and adult–child interactions become more and more like adult–adult interactions and thus arrive at the bottom of Figure 3.2. Many of us may choose to have a family at this stage and thus we return back to the top of Figure 3.2 but this time as caregivers.

This developmental progression of interactive alignments provides us with a framework for the study of the child's communicative development which will be returned to when children's acquisition of pragmatic ability is examined (Chapters 4, 5 and 6). It will also be useful as a basis for assessment and intervention (see Chapters 7 and 8).

Concluding remarks

In this chapter methods for studying pragmatic disability in children have been examined. These studies have mainly involved language-impaired children in comparison with children matched for chronological age and for stage of language development. The predicted outcome of these studies is that language-impaired children will be inferior to their age-matched peers in terms of pragmatic skills but will be similar to language-matched peers.

However, there are two problems with this prediction. On the one hand, several studies have come up with alternative findings. For example, some language-impaired children have been found to be superior to their language-matched peers in terms of pragmatic ability. These alternative findings require explanation. But, more seriously, there is the problem that the studies described here have started from the hypothesis that language ability and pragmatic ability are necessarily related – and, in particular, that language ability determines pragmatic ability. As suggested in Chapters 5 and 6, pragmatic ability needs to be considered in relation to other abilities and aspects of development – linguistic, cognitive, sociocognitive, and affective – in complex ways. Some of these relationships have been brought out in case studies and group comparison studies described in this chapter, but there is a need to pursue these relationships further.

Chapter 4
Pragmatic Ability in Children: Development and Disorders

In this chapter a review is given of the development of children's pragmatic ability and of disorders in their use of language. Results are presented from studies of "normally" developing children in order to provide a background and framework for discussion of disordered development. First the origins of communication in infancy are examined and then some of the necessary ingredients of communication – such as reciprocity and intentionality – are shown to have their origins in developments that take place in the first year of life.

Early communicative development

There have been numerous studies of communication between infants and their caregivers in the first year of life (see, for example, Schaffer, 1977; Lock, 1978; Bullowa, 1979). These studies have shown how some components of linguistic communication, such as reciprocal behavior, can be found in the prelinguistic stage, before children have acquired any language at all. More recently, there has been a focus on the question of continuity between the prelinguistic and subsequent linguistic stages, and, in particular, with the question of whether early communicative interactions provide a basis for the development of language and communication (Golinkoff, 1983a).

Infant–caregiver interaction and proto-conversations

Two distinct patterns of behavior have been identified in very early infant–caregiver interaction. In the first, the behaviors of infant and caregiver, which may consist of gestures and vocalizations, are closely synchronized, thus giving the impression of a closely coordinated activity (Trevarthen, 1979). The second pattern, which is more similar to later linguistic communication, involves reciprocal activity in which the participants take turns and the turns are complementary to one another.

For example, the mother smiles and then the baby smiles, or the baby smiles and then the mother talks, smiles or laughs (Whiten, 1977).

Some studies have shown how the infant takes the lead in these interactions. For example, it has been observed that during breast-feeding, where the mother jiggles during pauses in the child's sucking, it is the baby who controls the duration of the jiggling (Kaye, 1977). Other studies have focused on how caregivers regulate interaction with the baby, by responding selectively to the baby's gestures and vocalizations and by timing their own behaviors to coordinate with those of the baby (Miller and Byrne, 1984). In so doing, caregivers treat aspects of the baby's behavior as if they were attempts to communicate and fit their own behaviors to those of the baby to give the appearance of more mature conversational interaction. These early interactions have been referred to as *proto-conversations* (Bateson, 1975). Snow (1977) has examined such conver-sations over several stages between mothers and infants aged from 3 to 18 months and has shown how mothers respond to and attempt to elicit contributions from their babies which can be interpreted as if they were intentional communications, and how, as the babies matured, the mothers came to expect higher quality contributions from their babies. The following example shows how a mother responds to the burps, yawns, sneezes, and vocalizations of her 3-month-old baby and incorporates them into a proto-conversation (Snow, 1977, p.12):

Ann:	(smiles)
Mother:	Oh what a nice little smile
	Yes, isn't that nice?
	There
	There's a nice little smile
Ann:	(burps)
Mother:	What a nice little wind as well
	Yes, that's better, isn't it?
	Yes

Although many studies of infant–caregiver interaction have emphasized the skilled role that the caregiver plays in interpreting the child's actions and coordinating them into conversation-like routines, it is important to consider different patterns of interaction which occur at this stage and their role in subsequent communicative development. Infant–caregiver interaction does not always run smoothly. Indeed, in one study successful episodes, in which an infant's initial signals were understood by the mother, accounted for only 38 percent of all interactions initiated by the infant (Golinkoff, 1986). However, although the mothers failed in their initial attempts to interpret their children's intents, they tended to persevere in helping the children to communicate, with the result that the children often repaired their original signals by repeating, augmenting or replacing them. These negotiation episodes frequently resulted in successful outcomes, so that the child was able to learn what devices were more likely to work when attempting to communicate intent. Furthermore, as a subsequent analysis of successful episodes indicates, there are some factors that facilitate communication. These include the extent to which the child communicates intents involving topics already established in the discourse, an increasing use of more conventional signals, and the ability of the caregiver to interpret these signals (Golinkoff and Gordon, 1988). Both unsuccessful and successful episodes could play a role in the child's development of pragmatic skills. Negotiation episodes provide occasions for the child to repair previously unsuccessful attempts, while successful episodes create the expectation that communicative effort is usually worth expending. Together, these episodes enable the child to distinguish between which communicative devices do and do not work in conversational contexts.

Much of early communication is achieved through facial expressions, eye contact, gesture, posture, and vocalization. However, it is necessary to ask two questions about these early interactions:

- Are they true examples of an early ability to communicate or simply the result of rich interpretation on the part of analysts (as well as parents)?
- Do these early interactions provide a basis for subsequent conversational development?

Taking the first question, if the earlier definition of communication is applied (see Chapter 1) – which requires an intention to communicate and a belief that the receiver would recognize that intention – then the early proto-conversations described cannot count as communication from the infant's perspective. In fact, an important characterization of these interactions is that the mother is described as treating the contributions of the infant *as if* they were intentional. It is suggested that in so doing the mother provides a basis for the child's communicative development. Indeed, there has been considerable research on early routines in which mothers play games such as "peekabo" with their babies (Bruner, 1975). In these routines the infant learns to produce a behavior of a constant form, to expect a predictable response, and eventually to anticipate parts of the sequence of actions. Some of these behaviors are similar to those required in taking turns in conversation. Moreover, over the course of several months the mother appears to provide a scaffold on which the child can build its communicative skills.

This brings us to the second question. Do these early interactions really help? For example, it has been argued that similarities between the infant's behaviors in proto-conversations and those required in linguistic turn-taking are more apparent than real and that, rather than having any turn-taking knowledge the infant may simply be unable to listen and respond at the same time (Shatz, 1983a). Furthermore, as already indicated, there are some essential components of real communication which appear to be absent from the behaviors produced by infants in the earliest stages. To consider this question more fully, it is necessary briefly to review how communicative ability develops in the first year of life.

It has often been assumed that newly born babies are devoid of any basic social motivation and that their requirements are purely physiologic. However, recent studies suggest that neonates are biologically predisposed for communication from the moment of birth – they spend their waking time moving their limbs, changing their facial expressions, attending to people and objects around them, and vocalizing. In other words, they display behaviors such as adult-like facial expressions and they make various speech-like movements involving the lips and tongue (Trevarthen, 1979). Of course, this does not mean that infants use these behaviors to communicate intentionally at this stage – rather it indicates that the potential for developing communicative ability is present at birth (Richards, 1974).

Early communication between infants and caregivers has been described as "a cross-personal dialogue of affect" which provides a foundation for the development of linguistic dialogue (Dore, 1983, p.188). What this means is that, in early interactions with a caregiver, the infant develops a motivation towards persons that is essential for dialogue. Out of this dialogue of affective expressions the infant learns to construct systems of meaning as well as the intention to communicate these meanings. Furthermore, it seems that there is an intimate relationship between the infant's and the caregiver's behaviors, in that the infant's affective signals elicit and reinforce the adult's vocalizations, while the prosodic characteristics of adult speech to infants are attractive and perceptually salient for the infant (Fernald, 1984).

Pinpointing when an infant's behaviors can be reliably described as being intentionally communicative is difficult, although several studies provide useful guidelines. By the end of the first year children seem to have become aware that certain of their behaviors and gestures can be used to achieve goals interpersonally (Bates, 1979; Harding and Golinkoff, 1979). In particular, children of this age begin to combine attention to persons and objects, and to use persons to obtain objects out of reach or use objects to attract a person's attention. This integration of attention to objects and persons, together with the development of the notion of indirect causality which permits the child to recognize that the adult is an agent of action independent of the child's control, has been called *secondary intersubjectivity* (Trevarthen and Hubley, 1978). To illustrate, observations of a baby at 25 weeks showed that the baby displayed extreme interest in objects to the neglect of the mother, or else attended solely to the mother. By 45 weeks, however, the infant was able to integrate attention to mother and objects. Indeed, as the following example shows, a child aged 12 months combined attention to her mother with attention to an object in order to elicit an action from her mother (Bates, Camaioni and Volterra, 1975):

> C. is sitting on her mother's lap, while M. shows her the telephone and pretends to talk. M. tries to press the receiver against C's ear and have her "speak", but C. pushes the receiver back and presses it against her mother's ear. This is repeated several times. When M. refuses to speak into the receiver, C. bats her hand against M.'s knee, waits a moment longer, watches M.'s face, and then, uttering a sharp aspirated sound /hɑ/, touches her mother's mouth.

This sequence of actions by the child has been described by Bates, Camaioni and Volterra as *proto-imperatives*, because they are precursors of requests which involve the use of human agents to operate on or obtain objects.

While detailed descriptions such as these provide a useful basis for showing how children's behaviors become more communicative, they still do not address the question of whether the child's behaviors can be reliably taken as intentions to communicate. Two types of evidence are typically used to support attributions of intentionality. The first uses behavioral evidence. For example, if an infant persists with a behavior, either repeating or recoding the message in the absence of the adult's response, and then stops signalling once the adult responds, then there is good evidence for attributing communicative intent to the infant's behaviors (Greenfield, 1980; Golinkoff, 1983b).

The second type of evidence is more indirect and attempts to relate the origins of intentional communication to stages of early cognitive development in which cognitive milestones are taken as prerequisites for the development of components of intention. Harding (1983) conducted a study of infants from the age of 6 to 11 months in which she related Piagetian stages of cognitive development to the development of communication. The study began when the children were at Piaget's stage 3, which involves the knowledge of means–end relationships. At this stage the children were using communicative procedures, such as vocalizing, reaching, and looking, but they could not be reliably interpreted as intention and only appeared communicative because of the mother's reaction to them. At stage 4, which involves knowledge of objective causality, the infant was beginning to use communicative behaviors instrumentally as a means of obtaining objects. However, it was only at stage 5, when the child becomes aware of others as autonomous sources of action, that intentional communication can be more reliably inferred. At this stage the child attends both to mother and objects, looking back and forth between them, indicating an awareness that communication can be used to get a person's attention and then use that person to achieve a goal.

Thus attributions of intentionality are constrained by independent evidence concerning the child's cognitive abilities which underlie intentional communication.

To conclude this section, the relevance of this account of early communicative development to the study of pragmatic disability in children is looked at using three main points.

First, some essential components of communication – reciprocity, intentionality, and awareness of other persons as independent agents – have their origins in developments that take place during the first year of life. It will be important to look for signs of these components of communication in older children who are communicatively impaired. At the same time, it is possible to indicate important differences between early communication and the skills that develop later. There is an important distinction between communicative intention and communicative ability. While the intention to communicate is an essential prerequisite for communication to take place, effective communication also depends on the acquisition and use of many complex abilities – linguistic, cognitive and social. Related to this is the observation that full communicative understanding depends on the ability to reason accurately about the knowledge and beliefs of other conversational partners – what has been referred to as a "theory of mind". This ability does not appear to be well developed until around the age of 3 (Shatz, 1983a). This point is returned to in Chapter 6. So, in looking at early communicative development the origins of communication can be traced and a note made of which aspects still have to be acquired.

A second issue is that studies of early communication have a prognostic value because they can serve as indicators of possible subsequent difficulties in language acquisition and communicative development. Wetherby, Yonclas and Bryan (1989) compared the communicative profiles of preschool children with handicaps – including children with Down's syndrome, specific language impairments, and autism – with those of normal children functioning at the prelinguistic and one-word stages. In other words, the handicapped children were matched for stage of language development with the nonhandicapped children. One aspect in which differences occurred was in the proportion of communicative acts involving behavioral regulation and joint attention. Compared to the nonhandicapped children, one of the language-impaired and all of the autistic children displayed an excess of behavioral regulation acts and a deficiency of joint attention acts. Because a deficiency in social awareness is often cited as a characteristic of the communication of autistic children, the early identification of such problems could be of major prognostic value. Thus studies of early communication could provide a useful index of subsequent developments in language and communication.

Finally, it is important to consider the role of interaction with caregivers in a child's development. Mothers and other caregivers structure interactions with their infants and provide a foundation for subsequent developments. There is an extensive body of research that suggests that features of caregiver–child interaction are significant for the child's linguistic and communicative development. This question will be returned to in Chapter 5.

Children's pragmatic development: an overview

Most research on the development of pragmatic ability has been based on the viewpoint that this is an area that is worthy of study in its own right, and not, for example, in so far as it sheds light on the acquisition of syntactic constructions or other aspects of language structure. Consequently, most studies have tended to examine the nature of children's acquisition of pragmatic skills without attempting to relate these skills to the children's developing linguistic competence. Among the skills studied are: turn-taking, contextual variation in the use of speech acts, narratives, initiating conversational exchanges, recognizing and repairing communicative breakdown, presupposition, and pragmatic inferences (Ervin-Tripp and Mitchell-Kernan, 1977; Ochs and Schieffelin, 1979; McTear, 1985a). Taken together, these are the main topics which are discussed in textbooks on pragmatics (see, for example, Brown and Yule, 1983; Leech, 1983; Levinson, 1983; Stubbs, 1983; McLaughlin, 1984). These topics in are reviewed in this section, looking at findings from naturalistic as well as experimental studies. Findings on pragmatic disability relating to these particular aspects of language use are also reviewed.

Turn-taking

Successful conversational turn-taking has been described as a skilled activity based on an intricate set of rules involving linguistic and pragmatic knowledge (Sacks, Schegloff and Jefferson, 1974). Generally in conversation one participant speaks at a time and transitions between speakers are usually accomplished with a minimum of gap between turns as well as little overlapping between the speakers. Sacks, Schegloff and Jefferson suggest that conversational participants who wish to take the next turn do not wait until the current speaker stops talking, because otherwise there would be regular and noticeable gaps between turns. Similarly, they do not seem to depend solely on nonverbal or prosodic cues of turn completion – such as the speaker directing gaze at the listener or the use of a falling intonation contour – but anticipate the potential completion of the turn and begin at that point. The observation that many overlaps occur at transition-relevant positions – for example, at the point where the speaker's turn consists of a potentially complete syntactic structure, such as subject–verb–object – supports the view that next speakers anticipate the potential completion of a turn with precision timing and start talking no sooner and also no later than the appropriate point. For example:

A: That's an interesting house, <u>isn't it</u>?
B: <u>Do you</u> like it?
(Overlapped speech underlined)

Overlaps occur as the current speaker may opt to continue beyond the transition-relevant position. In this example, for instance, the first speaker adds a tag that continues the turn beyond its first transition-relevant position and the overlap occurs because the second speaker starts to speak at precisely this point. As we can see, turn-taking is a dynamic and locally managed activity as turn lengths are negotiated on a moment-by-moment basis at each transition-relevant position instead of being predetermined or agreed in advance.

Children's turn-taking

It has been suggested that the turn-taking of young children differs from the model proposed for adult turn-taking because they are unable to project possible turn completion points. Garvey and Berninger (1981) found that gaps between turns were longer for younger children (aged 2;10 to 3;3) than for older children (aged 4;7 to 5;7) and for adults. They also found few overlaps in the data for the younger children. Combining these findings, they concluded that young children may not rely so much on a projection of possible turn completion for deciding when it is their turn to talk as on cues, such as terminal intonation patterns, as well as on a brief interval of silence following their partner's speech.

This inability to process the turn in progress also results in more irrelevant next turns, particularly in multiparty talk or when attempting to intrude into an ongoing conversation – both situations which preschool children find difficult (Ervin-Tripp, 1979). By 3 or 4 years, however, children have the ability to repair overlaps by stopping when interrupted or by repeating the overlapped portions when interrupting, while by 4$ years they are already able to make explicit observations about turn-taking procedures and types of talk (Ervin-Tripp, 1979).

The ability to project possible turn completions appears to develop relatively early. Gallagher and Craig (1982) studied the simultaneous speech of 4-year-old girls in three-party conversations. They distinguished between sentence-initial overlaps, in which two speakers start a turn at the same time, and sentence-internal overlaps, in which the second speaker begins after the first speaker has said a few words. Sentence-initial overlaps involve breakdown in the turn exchange system which allocates rights of speaking to conversational participants. According to the model of Sacks, Schegloff and Jefferson (1974), the right of the current speaker to continue supersedes the listener's right to self-select unless the current speaker chooses not to continue and does not select the next speaker. Thus sentence-initial overlaps reflect social rules that may differ from one culture to another, or indeed from one speech event to another. Sentence-internal overlaps are more interesting for our present purposes, because they involve the integration of linguistic and pragmatic knowledge. Sentence-internal overlaps can be divided into two types: those in which the second speaker begins talking before the current speaker has reached a potential point of completion (in other word, interruptions), and those in which the second speaker attempts to project the turn completion but the current speaker continues beyond that transition-relevant position (i.e. overlaps). Gallagher and Craig found that the children they studied appeared to project turn completions, because overlaps occurred at positions where transition was relevant – such as at the completion of structures such as subject-transitive verb-object, subject-intransitive verb, or subject-(potentially)intransitive verb. The following example illustrates an overlap which occurs following a potentially intransitive verb (Gallagher and Craig, 1982, p.71):

A: I'm gonna eat a <u>cookie</u>
B: <u>Wanna</u> make more?

Similar examples are discussed in McTear (1985a).

Children's difficulties with turn-taking

Kysela et al. (1990) studied the turn-taking abilities of language-impaired children at the one-word utterance stage in comparison with language-matched younger children. Turn-taking is more primitive at the one-word stage because there is no scope for sentence-internal overlap, which is a more precise indicator of mature conversational turn-taking. In this study a turn was simply an action or communication by one person who stopped and waited for the other person to act or communicate. Each turn was coded by mode – motor-gestural action, vocalization, word, or phrase – and the turn-taking sequences were measured for extent of mode-matching, which is an indicator of primitive topic continuation. The turn-taking performance of the impaired dyads compared favorably with that of the comparison group dyads for number and length of mode-matched turn-taking sequences. This result indicates that language-impaired children were motivated to engage in contingent conversation. However, it is necessary to examine more sophisticated conversational turn-taking to see where problems arise due to the interaction of linguistic abilities and pragmatic factors.

Craig and Evans (1989) compared the turn-taking skills of five language-impaired children, aged 8;8 to 13;11, with those of five younger normal language children aged 2;9 to 3;9 matched for MLU and five chronologically age-matched normal language children aged 8;5 to 14;1.

Comparisons were made of the amount of simultaneous speech produced by each group and of turn-initial and turn-internal overlaps. It was found that the language-impaired children produced significantly less simultaneous speech than either normal language group. While this finding may appear counter-intuitive, as simultaneous speech is a possible indication of conversational breakdown and consequently more likely to be expected in interaction with language-impaired children, a closer examination of the subtypes of simultaneous speech reveals some interesting findings.

Sentence-initial overlaps, it will be recalled, occur when both adult and child begin to talk at the same time. They are examples of turn exchange errors, when both participants compete for the floor. Craig and Evans found that sentence-initial overlaps were functionally similar across subject groups.

The main differences were found with sentence-internal overlaps, which occur when one person starts to speak after the other person has said a few words but has not completed his or her turn. These overlaps can occur under two qualitatively quite different circumstances. On the one hand, the overlap may be due to an interruption, in which the second speaker begins without taking account of the turn in progress. The following example, in which overlapped words are underlined, illustrates an interruption in which the child interrupts with an utterance that is unrelated to what the adult is saying (Craig and Evans, 1989, p. 346):

Adult: Are you gonna make yours flat? (making a roof)
Child: Here's a guy (picks up a farm figure)

This example involved the introduction of new information by the child which was not related to the content of the adult's turn. In other cases the child continued with information that was a semantically related continuation of the child's previous utterances, again disregarding the adult's turn.

The second type of sentence-internal overlap results from the more sophisticated turn-taking behavior described earlier, in which the listener attempts to predict the completion of the current turn and starts to talk with an utterance that is semantically related to that turn. The following is an example (Craig and Evans, 1989, p. 346):

Adult: So you think you are going to do breaststroke or just
            freestyle?
Child: I haven't trained myself in breaststroke

This type of overlap is an indication of precision timing in which the child has to integrate pragmatic and linguistic knowledge in order to predict, on the basis of the utterance so far, how the utterance is likely to continue and when it will reach a possible completion point. Craig and Evans refer to these overlaps as "premature responses".

Table 4.1 Sentence-internal overlaps

Subject group	Premature response	Continuation	New
SLI	17	61	22
NL-A	80	17	3
NL-L	76	19	5

SLI=specifically language-impaired subjects
NL-A =normal language age-matched subjects
NL-L=normal language language-matched younger subjects
Based on Craig & Evans, 1989, p. 339

The findings from this study are illuminating, as indicated in Table 4.1. The sentence-internal overlaps of the language-impaired group were mainly continuations of previous utterances or new information – in other words, immature interruptions. The overlaps of both normal language groups, on the other hand, were mainly premature responses – that is, precision-timed overlaps occurring at transition relevant utterance positions. These results, along with other evidence concerning resolution of the overlaps and turn switch times, indicate that the turn-taking behaviors of the normal language groups were more sophisticated than those of the language-impaired children.

Turn-taking plays an important role in conversational management and is motivated by the need to maintain a smooth flow of conversation and an equitable distribution of turns. Sentence-initial overlaps provide evidence of breakdown of these aspects of turn-taking. The verbal characteristics of sentence-initial overlaps were similar across groups, with children continuing the meaning of a previous utterance and usually giving up the floor after a few overlapped words. As far as nonverbal characteristics were concerned, most of the overlaps were preceded by the children averting their gaze from the adult so that they were unable to monitor for turn exchange cues. As the results indicate, the language-impaired children were as proficient as the normal language groups in these conversational aspects of turn-taking.

Sentence-internal overlaps are different, however, because the ability to take the floor at a transition-relevant position requires the child to process the form and meaning of the adult's utterance in order to be able to predict a possible grammatical completion and to begin talking with semantically related information. In other words, linguistic ability is required. Craig and Evans suggest that the language-impaired children did not have the encoding and decoding skills necessary to take the floor at linguistically appropriate points in the conversation and that they seemed to be still processing previous sentence information when they interrupted. The following example illustrates how a child seems to be responding to the adult's first utterance while overlapping with part of the adult's continuation, thus appearing not to be processing the second part of the adult's turn at all (Craig and Evans, 1989, p. 346):

Adult: Do you need some more firemen?
            My guys <u>got his</u> mask on
Child: <u>No</u>

This link between linguistic ability and turn-taking is further supported when we consider that all of the premature responses (the more mature overlaps) of the language-impaired group were due to one child whose receptive language abilities were unimpaired. Thus a fine-grained analysis, using more elaborate measures of linguistic impairment, reveals the role played by linguistic knowledge in this aspect of turn-taking.

Initiating conversational exchanges

The ability to initiate conversational exchanges, for example, by asking questions, making requests or observations, involves social, cognitive, and linguistic skills. A child has to have the desire to initiate conversation spontaneously but also has to be able to design the initiation according to the needs of the listener and the situation. One aspect of pragmatic disability is a failure to initiate conversation; another is the use of inappropriate strategies for initiating. Consequently it is important to examine the development of initiating abilities in young children.

Children's initiations of conversational exchanges
In a study of relations between the utterances of young children and their mothers, Bloom, Rocissano, and Hood (1976) found that at first young children were more likely to respond to adult utterances than to initiate conversation. Similarly, Halliday (1975) located the onset of dialogue in his son Nigel at around 18 months but found that Nigel's interactional repertoire comprised mainly responses, with only "What's that?" questions being used to initiate dialogue.

Getting the listener's attention is a prerequisite for successful communication. Social knowledge is involved because the speaker must assess whether the attention of the listener has been obtained. Attention-getting devices can be both verbal and nonverbal and are used by children as young as 2 years (Wellman and Lempers, 1977). A range of attention-getting devices – including establishing eye contact, touching or approaching the addressee, vocatives and particles such as *hey* – have been illustrated in McTear (1985a).

In addition to getting the listener's attention, it is also necessary to structure the content of the initiating utterance so that the addressee's attention is appropriately directed to the persons, objects and events being discussed. Establishing a discourse topic involves making assumptions about what the addressee does and does not know, because referents that are new to the conversation and potentially unfamiliar to the addressee must be introduced differently from those that have already been established in the course of the conversation. So, for example, using a pronoun, as in "He hit me", or a definite article, as in "Where's the book?", is inappropriate if the addressee cannot locate the referents of *he* and *the book*. Thus attention-directing involves social and cognitive skills to enable the child to assess the state of the listener's knowledge, as well as linguistic skills, to know which linguistic form matches the situation.

The origins of attention-directing have been traced back to the prelinguistic stage where children use gestures coordinated with vocalizations to direct the addressee's attention to an object (Carter, 1978; Foster, 1986). Common nouns can also be used as an attention-directing strategy (Atkinson, 1979). For example, a child holding up a toy car and saying "Car" might not be labelling the object but drawing attention to it. Supporting evidence for this interpretation would be provided if once the adult had acknowledged attention, the child went on to predicate something about the object – for example, *broken*. This sort of interactionally constructed sequence has been widely reported and appears to precede a later stage in which the two words are linked syntactically in a single utterance (Scollon, 1976).

The devices that can be used for attention-directing vary according to the situation. In the context of reference to objects in the immediate environment, nonverbal devices such as pointing and showing can be used. Referents that are not in the immediate physical context require more elaborate verbal devices, such as relative clauses or attention-locating phrases such as "Do you know" or "Do you remember". In the following example, taken from McTear (1985a, pp. 81–2), a child (aged 5;1) is trying to identify for her friend an object – a birthday card – that she sent to her father. Although the object is in the present environment, it is out of reach and in a row including several other cards, so that simply pointing would probably be ineffective and other verbal devices such as locating the card with reference to its neighbor and describing the card are necessary:

> (*S goes to mantelpiece to point out the card*)
> S: See that see that very first one (points to card)
>   Just beside the racing car one?
> H: Uhhuh
> S: See that one with the little girl in <u>it</u>? (points)
> H: <u>That's</u> a little <u>car</u>

S: <u>See</u> this one (points)
H: I'll sh- I'll tell
S: No see that one (points)
H: That one? (points)
S: Uhhuh
      Well that is the one I gived him
(Parts of utterances that were spoken simultaneously are underlined).

As can be seen, establishing the referent involved the use of verbal and nonverbal devices. Moreover, in this case it required several attempts as well as some degree of collaboration from the other child.

It is useful to compare examples such as this with the findings reported in studies of referential communication. One aspect of these tasks is that a child has to describe an object – such as a picture – from a set of objects that differ in respect of certain criterial features. Another person, cast in the role of listener and separated from the speaker by a screen, has to select the correct object from an identical set of objects. For example, the pictures might be as follows:

– A man holding a flag pointed upwards and wearing a hat.
– A man holding a flag pointed downwards and wearing a hat.
– A man holding a flag pointing upwards with no hat.
– A man holding a flag pointing downwards with no hat.

Each picture is different and can be identified only on the basis of an accurate assessment and description of its criterial features. Generally young children have difficulty with such experimental tasks. In some cases they use devices such as pointing or deictic expressions such as *this*, which are inappropriate in the context of a listener unable to see what the speaker is referring to. In other cases the description is inadequate because it does not uniquely identify the picture (for example, *the man with a hat*). A further inadequacy may be the inclusion of unnecessary information – for example, a description of the man's jacket if all the pictures depict the same jacket (Whitehurst and Sonnenschein, 1981).

How can we explain these discrepant findings? One common explanation is in terms of task difficulty and artificiality. In some earlier experiments children were required to describe abstract shapes for which they lacked the appropriate vocabulary. As a result they tended to use inappropriate descriptions, including gestures and deictics, possibly as a strategy for communicating at least something to the listener. Moreover, many experimental tasks do not permit feedback from the listener, so that the speaker's message has to be correctly designed and produced with less opportunity to assess the listener's state of knowledge than is available in more natural situations. Thus children may be unaware of the listener's needs, or perceive the needs inaccurately, rather than being unable to design their message appropriately. In the earlier example, in which a child attempted to identify a birthday card, the feedback from the listener obviously helped the speaker to work towards an appropriate description.

However, experimental studies indicate with some precision those areas in which a child is lacking in skills. In the case of attention-directing, the skills involve a greater degree of abstraction than is normally required in conversational contexts, although these skills become important in school contexts as well as in conversations with other persons who do not share the child's world to the same extent as family and close friends. Experimental studies also indicate that children develop a more abstract concept of messages which will be necessary for the identification and resolution of communicative misunderstandings. For example, in experiments in which children observed a communicative episode containing some messages that were purposely designed to be inadequate, young children aged 5 tended to blame the listener for the communication problem, while older children were able to identify the source of the problem in the speaker's message (Robinson and Robinson, 1977).

To conclude this section, children's re-initiations, which occur when either no response or an unsatisfactory response has been received, are examined. Re-initiations are interesting because they provide evidence that the child is actively pursuing a response – thus disconfirming the hypothesis that the utterances of young children are largely egocentric. Re-initiations can also be examined for the range of linguistic devices used to obtain a more satisfactory response.

Children display an ability to re-initiate from an early age. Halliday (1975) reports that at age 9 months his son used a loud, more intensified form to express the meaning "do that again" when his first attempt failed to elicit a response. By 15 months the child was using intonation to distinguish a re-initiated form. In a naturalistic study of 2 year olds, Wellman and Lempers (1977) found that the children re-initiated 54 percent of the time following no response, often adapting the original message to include more initiating devices such as attention-getting words, vocatives and eye contact. Similar findings are reported by McTear (1985a).

Re-initiations can involve either a repetition of the preceding utterance or a rephrasing. Rephrasings indicate greater flexibility, although even utterances that are repeated verbatim may be modified prosodically. The following is an example from McTear (1985a, p. 92) in which a combination of devices is used to gain a response:

(S is talking about an alarm clock)
S: That's what can wake you up very hard early in the mornings
      Um it could
      Couldn't it daddy?
      Couldn't that one daddy?

Could that sort – couldn't that sort of one wake you up very early?
F: Umhmm

In summary, children use a variety of devices to get and direct their listener's attention. They are also able to use similar devices to re-initiate when they are initially unsuccessful. Young children who are unimpaired communicatively would seem to be motivated to initiate conversational exchanges from an early age – even before language is acquired. However, the ability to perform these initiations appropriately only develops gradually over a period of time during the preschool and early school years, their initiations becoming more sophisticated as they develop a greater awareness of their listener's needs and a repertoire of the linguistic devices required.

Difficulties with conversational initiations
Impairment of conversational initiations can take several different forms. The following examples, taken from the case study of McTear (1985b), illustrate some aspects. The child in this study had been described as being fairly responsive in conversation, in that he tended to provide at least a minimal and appropriate response to questions, though he adopted a mainly noninitiating role, so that the task of maintaining the conversation was left to his dialogue partner. In the first extract, in which he was describing a hotel in which he had stayed, the child appears to recognize the social obligation to take a turn but is unable to contribute any meaningful content and fills out by producing gradually reduced repetitions of his previous utterances:

Child:	It's got twenty windows in it
Adult:	Um
Child:	It has rooms. It has. It has a lift
Adult:	Um
Child:	In it
	(2.0)
	has a lift in it
	(1.2)
	lift in it
Adult:	How long did you stay there for?

In the next extract the child is involved in a communicative task in which he has to describe what he would do in a set of problem situations. Prior to this particular example, he had been discussing a picture in which a boy had been locked out of his house and the different actions that the boy could take. Different actions were portrayed on cards and the child discussed these adequately – for example, the boy could climb in through an open window, telephone his mother, or wait for her outside the house. One action involved going to a neighbor's house. Following an interchange that established that the child understood the situation, the investigator asked the child what he thought the boy might say to the neighbor:

Adult:	And what's he saying to that lady?
Child:	Hello
Adult:	Yes, and what do you think he'll say next?
Child:	Nice to see you
Adult:	Uhhuh
	But do you remember then as well he's lost his key and can't get in
	So what's he going to tell her
Child:	I've lost my key
	He might say: where's my key
	Did anybody see my key?
Adult:	Right

As we can see, the child is able to put himself in the role of the boy in the picture and imagines what the boy might say. However, the initial exchanges are odd – he greets the woman and makes a polite comment, but has to be prompted to come up with the appropriate message. In comparison, a normally developing child of the same age, when asked what she would say in this situation, replied "Excuse me – I've lost my key and my mummy and daddy are out".

In isolation these examples are not particularly remarkable; however, they are typical of many similar interactions with the child, in which he failed to take an initiating role in conversation and was content to keep the talk at the level of polite niceties. The first example may suggest an inability to organize a description in such a way as to present information that is useful and interesting to a listener. Similarly, in the second example, he seems to lose track of the main point of the situation and thus fails to produce an informative message. What is not clear is whether the child has a primary difficulty in organizing extended discourse – such as a description or a narrative – or in adapting it to the needs of his listeners. Whatever the cause, we can see how his ability to play more than a responsive role in conversation by taking the initiative and producing relevant and appropriate messages is seriously impaired.

A child may be unresponsive in social interaction, either through unwillingness or inability to initiate conversational exchanges. Autistic children, for example, have often been reported as initiating less frequently than other language-impaired children, thus indicating that they may lack communicative intent in addition to other linguistic and communicative disabilities. It has also been reported that many language-impaired children seem to have difficulty in playing an active role in conversation – that, for example, they ask very few questions (Morehead and Ingram, 1976; Kamhi and Johnston, 1982). However, it is important to take contextual factors into account, such as the child's motivation in the conversational task or his or her relationship with the listener. For example, it was found in one study that language-impaired children adopted a mainly nonassertive role when interacting with partners who were linguistically more advanced, but became more assertive when interacting with children who were linguistically less adept than themselves (Fey, Leonard and Wilcox, 1981).

Some of these contextual factors were examined in a recent study of the conversational responsiveness and assertiveness of language-impaired children (Rosinski-McClendon and Newhoff, 1987). Ten language-impaired children aged 4;1 to 5;9 were matched for MLU with 10 nonimpaired children and examined using samples of free conversation with an adult into which systematic probes were inserted. These probes consisted of questions to test the children's responsiveness; failures to respond to the children's initiations; and changes of topic by the experimenter to test their assertiveness – by, for example, continuing with the topic despite the absence of response or by re-introducing the original topic in the face of the changed topic. The language-impaired children were less responsive than their language-matched peers as measured by the extent to which they answered questions verbally. However, they proved to be equally assertive in comparison with the nonimpaired children in the measures of conversational assertiveness. Following no response by the listener, both groups tended to assert themselves by repeating their request. When the listener attempted to change the topic, however, both groups were minimally assertive and tended to follow the adult's lead. Interpreting these results, Rosinski-McClendon and Newhoff suggest that the reduced responsiveness of the language-impaired children to the experimenter's questions may have been the result of syntactic or semantic comprehension deficits rather than of a pragmatic disability, because the children were as assertive as their normal language peers in the conversational skills of topic maintenance and re-introduction. In other words, the language-impaired group did not appear to be qualitatively deficient in their use of language; rather their reduced responsiveness was a consequence of their linguistic deficiencies. Thus this study supports the earlier argument that it is necessary to separate out linguistic, cognitive and social aspects of language use in order to explain pragmatic disability. Similar indirect influences of syntactic and semantic deficits on the failure of language-learning-disabled children to produce questions spontaneously and to adopt defensive strategies in conversation have been investigated in several studies, the results of which are summarized and discussed in Donahue (1987).

Even if a child is prepared to initiate conversational exchanges, the initiations may be inappropriate – for example, they may be performed without the use of a required attention-getting device or with inadequate specification of the objects mentioned in the utterance. Autistic children often fail to use attention-getting devices such as establishing eye contact or vocatives (Fay and Schuler, 1980). They also tend to use questions excessively and inappropriately, not as a means of obtaining information but rather of eliciting a response, regardless of any topical relevance (Hurtig, Ensrud and Tomblin, 1982). Likewise, Baltaxe (1977) reports a tendency in adolescents to ask the same question over and over again, despite receiving an answer. These deficiencies in initiating do not appear to be related to any linguistic deficits; rather they would seem to be the result of an inability to produce talk that is appropriate to the current context.

The ability to produce informative messages has been investigated widely in studies of children's referential communication. Language-learning-disabled children appear to be less proficient than nondisabled peers in providing informative and communicatively effective messages when describing ambiguous figures or geometric shapes to a listener (Noel, 1980; Lloyd and Beveridge, 1981; Spekman, 1981; King, 1989). As with many similar studies, it is difficult to separate out the possible effects of linguistic deficits from an inability to adopt the listener's perspective. However, the children in these studies had not been identified as having specific linguistic difficulties. Moreover, their descriptions were qualitatively different from those of the nondisabled children: they were unable to provide discriminating information, tended to omit critical attributes or to place them at the end of their messages rather than in a more prominent position, and were less likely to describe the overall pattern of the referent but instead described its isolated parts. Thus these children seem unable to realize which sort of description would be more likely to ease the identification process for a listener – in other words, they appear to have a difficulty in assessing the listener's perspective.

Drawing a listener's attention appropriately to the referents of the discourse and introducing new topics in conversation appear to pose problems for autistic children who have been reported as being unable to distinguish between old and new information with a resultant usage of odd intonation patterns and a misuse of anaphoric pronouns, definite articles, and relative pronouns (Baltaxe, 1977); a tendency to over-specify discourse referents so that speech is often redundant (Fay and Schuler, 1980); and a failure to introduce new topics appropriately, for example, by using phrases such as *by the way* (Fay and Schuler, 1980). Similarly, Greenlee (1981) noted in her case study how her subject had problems in establishing discourse referents. In each of these cases the children had already developed the required linguistic structures but were using them inappropriately, so that their pragmatic disability was distinct from their level of linguistic development – indeed, their odd linguistic productions were the effect of, rather than the cause of, a qualitative pragmatic disability.

Speech acts

Speech acts are ways of doing things with words, such as making requests, promises, statements, or asking questions. Speech act theory is concerned with how language is used to accomplish these sorts of speech acts. Thus the emphasis is on the functions of language, on how language is used to achieve communicative goals in conversation (Searle, 1969). More specifically, speech act theory has examined the conditions under which a speech act is appropriately performed – for example, what it takes for a speaker to intend to make a promise and for a listener to recognize that intention, and how promises are different from other speech acts such as warnings or threats. Consequently, speech acts can be seen to involve several sorts of knowledge relevant for communication:

– linguistic knowledge of how particular structures can be used to perform certain functions;
– social knowledge of the contextual considerations that determine the appropriate situations for the use of a speech act;
– sociocognitive knowledge that guides the choice of a particular form of a speech act on the basis of perceived characteristics of the listener.

Requests are a good example of an instrumental use of language that involves an integration of these different types of knowledge. Making a request involves not only indicating clearly to a listener what action is desired; in order to maximize the chances of getting the listener to comply with the request the speaker needs to take into account the current situation, the speaker's and the listeners' roles and status, and the listeners' needs and purposes – in other words, getting another person to do what one wants is a complex, social, communicative skill (Becker, 1982, 1990; Bruner, Roy and Ratner, 1982).

Children's speech acts: requests

The origins of children's requesting strategies can be found in prelinguistic behaviors in the first year of life when gestures and vocalizations can be interpreted with some reliability from about the age of 9 months as intentional requesting schemata (Carter, 1978). During the second year requests are realized by combinations of gestures with names of desired objects and words such as *more, want,* and *gimme,* while by the third year children are using more elaborate forms such as embedded imperatives (for example, "Would you push this?") (Read and Cherry, 1978). By the age of 4 children are using request strategies that involve several steps for their successful accomplishment, and by the age of 5 or 6 they can use hints that do not specify the required goal (for example, "She's not letting me play with the doll's house"). As they move into school age, children learn more effective strategies for persuasion, such as reasons for the request or justifications directed towards the listener's social rights and desires (Garvey, 1975; McTear, 1985a). From about age 8 children's requesting strategies become even more sophisticated as they begin to recognize that requests intrude on the listener and so they become sensitive to the costs to the listener in their formulation of requests and acknowledge options for noncompliance (Mitchell-Kernan and Kernan, 1977). For reviews of the development of children's requesting strategies, see Becker (1982, 1990), Ervin-Tripp (1977), Ervin-Tripp and Gordon (1984), and McTear (1985a).

One of the more interesting findings from studies of children's requests is that the children appear from an early age to adapt their requests to social features of the speech situation, in particular to their perceptions of the social status of their listeners. Ervin-Tripp (1977) reviewed several studies that showed how children as young as 2 years differentiated age and rank of listener by addressing simple imperatives to peers, but desire statements, question directives and permission directives to adults. Similarly, Bates (1976) found that children aged between 3 and 6 years were able to modify their request forms in order to make them more polite, and were able to make judgments about degrees of politeness in requests in a comprehension task. However, the ability to draw on linguistic and sociocognitive knowledge and to make explicit reference to the pragmatic rules used when making judgments of politeness does not appear to develop until around the age of 7 (Baroni and Axia, 1989). Indeed, Garton and Pratt (1990) found that the ability of children to distinguish between the dimensions of politeness, effectiveness and likelihood of use of particular request forms was still developing between the ages of 8 and 12. Taken together, these findings would suggest that children have much greater social sensitivity than would be predicted from Piaget's theory of childhood egocentrism and from studies of children's role-taking abilities in experimental settings.

Levin and Rubin (1983) investigated the relationships between children's requesting strategies and their role-taking abilities in order to find an explanation for this discrepancy. They found a developmental progression in children's ability to use indirect requests, to formulate requests in such a way as to anticipate a successful outcome, and to use flexible re-initiation strategies when faced with noncompliance (see also McTear, 1985a). However, they found only limited support for a relationship between these requesting behaviors and independent measures of the children's role-taking abilities. Thus it may be that, in making requests, children are attuned to the more salient characteristics of listeners, such as age, sex and dominance status, but not necessarily to more fine-grained characteristics such as the listener's beliefs and intentions. In other words, the skills required for effective requesting may depend on more global role-taking as well as on strategies learned through previous experience rather than on a highly developed "theory of mind". It will be useful to consider this distinction when the difficulties some children have with the use of appropriate request forms are examined.

It is also illuminating to go beyond the analysis of requests as isolated speech acts and to examine how children negotiate requests over extended sequences of conversation. Requests are prime examples of goal-directed behavior and it is to be expected that a child who makes a request might persist if the initial response is noncompliant until compliance is achieved or is seen to be unlikely. Likewise, a requestee might have different goals and intentions from the requester and might wish to persist with refusing to comply with the request. McTear (1985a) examined request sequences involving two preschool girls and found that the children's devices for re-initiating requests and for expressing noncompliance became more sophisticated with age. Initially, the children tended to simply repeat their requests, but as they developed they would often rephrase the request, in some cases using more polite forms, in other cases more aggravated forms, and would provide justifications for the request and counter-arguments to the other child's justifications of her reasons for rejecting the request. Similarly the child rejecting the request would initially refuse with simple forms such as *no*, but later would justify the refusal or provide a counter-argument to the other child's justification for the request. Thus the children moved from rigid to more flexible strategies, with an increasing ability to justify their requests and refusals and to take account of their partner's objections and justifications.

The comprehension of requests also provides us with useful inform-ation about a child's ability to recognize another person's intentions, particularly in the case of indirect requests in which the requested action is not stated explicitly. One surprising finding is that children as young as 2 years can respond appropriately to requests such as "Can you find me a car?" or "Are there any more sweeties?" (Shatz, 1978). However, as Shatz showed, young children seem to operate with an action-based rule that leads them to interpret utterances such as these as requests for action even in contexts where an interpretation as a request for information is more appropriate. Nevertheless, Reeder (1980) found that children aged 2;6 to 3;0 were able to discriminate offers from requests in utterances that were worded ambiguously (for example, "Would you like to play on the bicycle?"). The ability to respond appropriately to direct and indirect requests appears to be closely related to comprehension ability, as shown in a study of the sensitivity of preschool children to the structure and linguistic complexity of requests (Ledbetter and Dent, 1988). Looking at older children, Ackerman (1978) examined how 6 and 8 year olds, as well as adults, interpreted utterances that could either be biased towards a literal meaning (e.g. a statement or a question) or a request, depending on the preceding context. It was found that both groups of children, as well as the adults, were able to make contextually sensitive interpretations of indirect speech acts, although this ability was less developed in the 6 year olds. Thus studies of children's comprehension of indirect requests suggests that children develop the ability to infer a speaker's intent based on an analysis of the form of an utterance and the context in which it was uttered.

Other speech acts

Children's production and comprehension of other types of speech acts has been less well documented. One recent study examined children's use of commissives – that is, utterances such as promises which commit the speaker to a certain course of action (Astington, 1988). Commissives appear to be a late development, because they have not been reported in studies of preschool children's speech acts. What is required in a commissive is that the speaker expresses an intention to perform some act in the future that will be of benefit to the listener, and furthermore that the speaker realizes that the expression of this intention is a commitment to this future action. Using a role-playing game in which the aim was to elicit an undeniably commissive speech act, Astington found that by about the age of 5 children are able to produce commissive speech acts, although it is only later that they are fully aware that the use of explicit performative words such as *promise* serves to reassure the listener that they are committed. In a subsequent study (Astington, 1990), children's judgments of whether different speech acts presented in a series of stories were examples of promising indicated that younger children were unable to distinguish between promising, in which the speaker has control of the future event, and predicting, in which the speaker does not usually have control. For example: saying "It will be a nice day tomorrow" should be interpreted as a prediction because the speaker cannot control the event, whereas saying "I'll bring it tomorrow" is a promise. It was only after the age of 9 that children could reliably distinguish between predictions and promises. Moreover, younger children's judgments were also biased by the outcome of the story. For example, they would tend to judge an act as a promise if the promise were subsequently fulfilled, but not if it turned out to be broken.

Another type of speech act that has been studied is expressives. Expressives function as routines in social interaction. Examples are saying "thank you", "you're welcome" and "I'm sorry" in the appropriate contexts. More complex examples are culturally determined routines such as the trick or treat routine at Halloween (Gleason and Weintraub, 1976).

Although parents begin to train their children in the appropriate use of these routines from an early age, it appears that many expressives are difficult to explain or justify to young children and that it is only at a later age that children fully understand their role in interpersonal communication.

Finally, there has been some research into the early development of children's ability to provide explanations. Previous work in developmental psychology, based in the Piagetian tradition, has emphasized the cognitive processes involved in explanation and has indicated that explanation is a relatively late acquisition because it involves the ability to understand and relate causal connections between two events. Within this tradition Donaldson (1986) has shown that children aged 3;6 to 4 can produce explanations in contexts that are familiar to them. However, explanations can also be used with the social function of regulating behavior – for example, giving a reason for a request or justifying an assertion. Taking this more social view of explanations, Barbieri, Colavita and Scheuer (1990) found that children as young as 3 years were able to produce different types of explanation and were sensitive to contextual and pragmatic constraints governing the act of explanation. For example, they were able to produce "why" type explanations when soliciting help from their listener to carry out a plan or when indicating that their partner's actions were undesired.

In summary, work to date on children's production and comprehension of speech acts indicates that a wide range of pragmatic factors is involved including: knowledge of the contextual conditions that make a particular speech act appropriate and of the communicative functions served by specific speech acts; knowledge of the characteristics of the listener that govern the choice of content and form of a speech act. The developmental trend, which is paralleled in other levels of language, is that children are able to produce and comprehend speech acts before they can make accurate judgments on usage. Furthermore, young children are often misled in comprehension and judgment tasks because they attend to surface features such as the form of the utterance or its outcome rather than to more complex contextual and pragmatic information such as the preceding discourse or the distinguishing features of the specific speech act. This tendency will also be discussed presently when dealing with how children make judgments concerning inadequate messages and inconsistencies in stories.

Difficulties with speech acts

Some studies have shown that language-impaired children have a more restricted range of speech acts than their normal language peers. However, counting the number of different speech acts a child uses or the number of times a particular speech act is used tells us little about how the child is using speech acts. Two aspects are particularly important: whether the child can interpret the intention expressed by an utterance, especially when the literal meaning is not the intended one, and whether the child is aware of the appropriate use of speech acts in different conversational contexts. The first aspect involves the comprehension of direct and indirect speech acts, while the second involves the ability to produce a particular linguistic form that is appropriate to the situation, including the task at hand and the social characteristics of the addressee, or to make judgments about the appropriacy of a speech act used by another person.

It has frequently been reported that some language-impaired children tend to take language too literally. For example, if they hear an utterance such as "Can you open the door", they will interpret it as a question, which is the literal interpretation, rather than as a request for action, which is the indirect meaning. Shatz, Bernstein and Shulman (1980) examined the responses of language-impaired children aged 5 and 6 years to indirect requests under two experimental settings and compared the findings with those of an earlier study of 2-year-old normal language children (Shatz, 1978). In the first condition the children heard several sentences, such as "Can you fit the ball in the truck?" or "The ball fits in the truck", which had more than one possible interpretation – either as a request for action or as a request for information. As in the earlier study it was found that the children's responses were almost entirely action responses – that is, the children used the simple strategy of responding with an action if such an action was possible. In the second condition, a prior linguistic context was established which would bias the interpretation one way or the other. For example, the experimenter would ask a series of unambiguous information questions, such as "Who talks on the telephone in your house?" and "Does mommy talk on the telephone?", and then produce a test utterance such as "Can you talk on the telephone?", which is ambiguous out of context but more likely to be intended as a request for information given the context of the previous utterances. The more linguistically sophisticated of the normal 2 year olds in the earlier study were sensitive to context and tended to produce fewer action responses in the contexts supporting informational responses. The language-impaired children, in contrast, appeared less able to generate informing responses, even when answering the unambiguous prior context sentences. They also seemed to have problems in taking the prior linguistic context into account. Thus the language-impaired children were deficient in their comprehension of indirect requests compared to their language-matched peers. This deficiency would appear to be attributable to their limited capacity to process prior linguistic information and integrate it into a coherent conversation.

Understanding what is involved in producing an appropriate speech act involves a combination of linguistic and social knowledge. The child must have available a repertoire of linguistic forms to express the particular speech act, must be able to distinguish listener attributes such as status and social distance, and must be able to choose the appropriate linguistic form to match the perceived listener attributes.

In one comparison study, Prinz (1982) examined the comprehension and production of requests by language-impaired children and language-matched peers. Although there were few differences on the comprehension task, it was found that the requests of the impaired group were less complete syntactically and phonologically. Furthermore, this group was less successful in a task that involved making judgments about the politeness of requests. However, it was not clear whether the deficiencies of these children were related to their impaired linguistic abilities or to an inability to perceive differences in the attributes of their listeners and to modify their requests accordingly.

These issues were investigated in a study of the requesting strategies of language-learning-disabled children and age-matched peers in a role-playing situation in which the children had to make requests of listeners differing in age or social status (Donahue, 1981). The children's requests were coded for politeness and persuasiveness. It was expected that the linguistic and social deficiencies of the language-learning-disabled group would result in a restricted ability to adjust their utterances according to differences in their listeners. Contrary to expectation, it was found that, compared with their normally achieving peers, the language-learning-disabled girls produced more polite requests and more persuasive appeals, while the language-learning-disabled boys used a range of linguistic forms to indicate politeness similar to normally achieving boys and were able to adjust the forms of their requests to reflect listener features. However, the language-learning-disabled boys made politeness adjustments according to power differences, while their normally achieving peers adjusted according to intimacy. Furthermore, the language-learning-disabled boys were actually more polite to lower-power than to higher-power listeners and used a smaller variety of persuasive appeals as well as fewer appeals requiring more advanced levels of listener perspective-taking. What these findings suggest is a deficiency in social understanding. The language-learning-disabled boys had an adequate linguistic repertoire and were able to make distinctions between listeners when making requests, but were unaware of the implications of these distinctions for socially appropriate speech.

Further evidence that language-learning-disabled children have difficulty in making socially appropriate adjustments in their speech was provided in a study of adjustments in communicative style when explaining a task to peers and younger listeners (Bryan and Pflaum, 1978). Compared to normal age-matched peers, language-learning-disabled boys appeared insensitive to audience differences in age in that they did not provide more instructions for younger listeners. Taken together, these studies indicate the need to control carefully for levels of linguistic and social knowledge and to understand the interdependence of these knowledge sources in the communicative use of language.

Clarification requests and the resolution of conversational misunderstandings

Resolving conversational breakdown depends on an ability to recognize when and in what way a message is inadequate and to know what steps need to be taken to repair the message. Studies of children's pragmatic abilities in naturalistic contexts have examined the extent to which children produce and respond appropriately to clarification requests (or contingent queries). In many cases the focus is on the interactional properties of clarificatory sequences – that is, the role played by both participants in the resolution of the problem. Experimental studies have examined the same phenomenon, with the main focus on the ability of children to recognize and respond to inadequate or ambiguous messages. Other related work deals with comprehension monitoring – that is, the ability to realize when you do not understand something. Generally the results from these different research traditions have presented conflicting pictures. In naturalistic studies children display remarkable competence in their production and comprehension of clarification requests, while in experimental studies their performance is less adequate. Some studies from both traditions will be examined and some conclusions drawn regarding these discrepancies.

Naturalistic studies

One of the earliest studies of children's use of and responses to clarification requests in a naturalistic context was by Garvey (1977). Garvey distinguished between several different types of clarification request and the responses they were intended to elicit. Some examples are:

1. Neutral or nonspecific request for repetition, e.g.

A: I want to play with the Lego
B: What?
A: I want to play with the Lego

2. Request for confirmation, e.g.

A: I want to play with the Lego
B: You want to play with the Lego?
A: Yes

3. Request for specific information, e.g.

A: I want to play with the Lego
B: Which Lego?
A: The big Lego

Garvey studied 48 children, aged 2;10 to 5;7, in dyadic peer interaction and found that they usually responded appropriately to the different types of clarification request and were also able to make appropriate requests for clarification. Similar findings are reported in McTear (1985a).

Several studies have examined the ability of younger children to respond to clarification requests in adult–child dialogues. Gallagher (1977) examined the responses of children aged 1;8 to 2;11 to neutral queries (requests for repetition) and found that they responded appropriately about 80 percent of the time. The children's revision strategies increased in variety with increase in language age. In a later study the responses of children aged 1;11 to 3;0 to the three types of query listed earlier were examined (Gallagher, 1981). The children were grouped according to the language developmental stages I, II and III (Brown, 1973). All of the children were able to respond appropriately to neutral queries and requests for confirmation, but only some of the children – those at stages II and III – were able to produce distinctive responses to requests for specific information. Thus it would seem that requests for specific information are more difficult and that the ability to respond appropriately to these requests is a later acquisition.

The acquisition of the ability to distinguish neutral and specific requests for clarification was studied by Anselmi, Tomasello and Acunzo (1986). The children were at language stages II–V. All of the children were able to differentiate between the two query types. Responses to neutral queries were usually repetitions of the entire utterance while in responses to specific queries the children replied with the requested information only. This finding is particularly interesting because it suggests that children have the pragmatic ability to modify their utterance according to the listener's needs, by supplying the information that the listener requires and omitting other information of which the listener is probably already aware. In other words, children's responses to specific queries suggest that they have some ability to assess their listener's state of knowledge and modify their utterances accordingly.

Most studies of children's responses to clarification requests examine single request–response exchanges. In order to respond to a series of requests a child would need to consider whether different types of response were required. The ability to respond to "stacked" requests was studied by Brinton et al. (1986). The children, whose ages ranged from 2;7 to 9;10, were assigned to four groups according to age level. The experimental task involved the children describing pictures to an examiner who was seated behind a screen. Some of the pictures were selected for initiation of a stacked request sequence, in which the examiner would respond to the child's initial description with "Huh?", to the child's response with "What?", and to the child's next response with "I didn't understand that". The children's response types were categorized as repetition, revision (paraphrase), addition (new information added), and cue (definition of term or explanation of background context). Several interesting findings emerged from this study. There was an age-related increase in the use of more sophisticated responses (i.e. not simple repetitions) as well as a decrease in inappropriate responses. The most advanced strategy – the use of cues – was produced only by the oldest age group, which suggests that by this age children have developed a wide variety of repair strategies and the ability to identify quite specifically the source of communicative breakdown. Finally, it was found that all groups used less repetition across stacked request sequences – that is, they frequently responded with a repetition to "Huh?", less frequently with a repetition to "What?", and even less frequently to the third request. Thus the children were able to revise their responses over the course of a request sequence, which suggests that they were responsive to the need to adapt their utterances to the requirements of their listeners.

Making a clarification request requires the ability to recognize that communicative breakdown has occurred as well as the ability to produce an appropriate query to elicit a repair. In a study of the emergence of clarification requests in children aged 1;6 to 3;0, Johnson (1980) found that requests for confirmation emerged at age 1;6, although the frequencies were small and many examples were unclear because the children often appeared to be simply echoing their mother's utterances using rising intonation and not necessarily attempting to request confirmation. Requests for confirmation emerged by age 2;2, while more specific requests were produced only by the older children. A similar developmental sequence was found by Gallagher (1981) who also reported a low frequency of child-initiated queries to adults compared with the numbers produced by adults to the children.

Experimental studies
Experimental studies have tended to support the view that children are poor at recognizing and repairing inadequate messages. In one study it was reported that children, whose ages ranged from 5;6 to 11;8, were presented with ambiguous messages and only requested clarification about half of the time, despite having been instructed to ask questions when the message was unclear (Ironsmith and Whitehurst, 1978). Taking this finding in conjunction with the reports from the studies of Johnson (1980) and Gallagher (1981) that young children infrequently initiated clarification request sequences, two conclusions are possible:

1. Children expect adults to formulate messages adequately and are reluctant to indicate otherwise.
2. Children are poor at recognizing when messages are inadequate or when they have failed to comprehend.

In order to investigate the first hypothesis, studies are needed which compare children's clarification requests to adult and child partners. At present there is only indirect evidence from naturalistic studies in the form of studies of children's clarification requests in peer interaction, where it has been found that children are capable of recognizing and repairing communicative breakdown (Garvey, 1977; McTear, 1985a). Some evidence has also been provided by an experimental study that showed that children react differently to ambiguous messages given by an adult or a peer – by incorrectly evaluating the adult's ambiguous utterance as informative, but correctly evaluating the peer's utterance (Sonnenschein and Whitehurst, 1980). A related hypothesis is that children expect adults to be cooperative and knowledgeable conversational partners and assume that the adult's message is informative. This hypothesis has been confirmed in experiments in which children had to select pictures based on an adult experimenter's descriptions (Jackson and Jacobs, 1982; Bredart, 1984). For example, there might be three pictures, one of a child with a stool, one of a child with a stool and a basin, and one of a child with an umbrella and a basin. If the message is "It's the child with the stool", then the first two pictures are potential referents and the child ought to ask for clarification in order to determine the correct referent. However, if the child is observing Grice's quantity maxim (Grice, 1975), which instructs a speaker to be informative enough and no more informative than necessary, then only the first picture (the child with the stool) is referenced by the message. Children appear to follow this maxim. Indeed, in Bredart's study, the children also provided justifications for their selections, such as "If it was this one, you would have said a stool and a basin". It will be important to consider these pragmatic aspects of children's responses as well as their different expectations of adult as opposed to child partners when the clarification requests of language-impaired children are examined below.

Turning now to the second hypothesis, it should be noted that there are some problems in the investigation of naturally occurring clarification sequences. First, they do not occur very frequently (for example, as few as 1 percent of the children's utterances in one of McTear's sampling stages). In any case, the absence of clarification requests may be a result of a lack of the need to seek clarification, because the children have learned to avoid communicative breakdown in the first place, rather than because of an inability to recognize and repair breakdown. Consequently, it becomes difficult to assess reliably whether children are able to recognize and respond to inadequate messages in naturally occurring conversation.

Moreover, there is no control over the utterances that might give rise to a clarification request – for example, except in a few clear-cut cases it is not possible to judge when an utterance ought to have been followed by a request for clarification and so to judge the extent to which children make the requests as required. There is a need for more detailed investigation of structural and pragmatic characteristics of the utterances for which clarifications are requested and their relationships to the types of request and response that they occasion (Furrow and Lewis, 1988). For these reasons, it is necessary to examine experimental studies of children's responses to ambiguous and inadequate messages in which there is more control over communicative breakdown.

Experiments designed to test children's ability to deal with ambiguous or inadequate information usually involve tasks in which the child has to select a picture or object from an array based on the experimenter's description. In some cases the description will not be sufficient to identify the referent uniquely. For example, if there are several pictures of a man, including one in which the man has a red flower and another in which he has a blue flower, then the description "a man with a flower" would not suffice to distinguish the two pictures. On recognizing this problem the listener should indicate that the message is inadequate.

Typically young children perform poorly in such tasks. Ironsmith and Whitehurst (1978) tested children whose mean ages ranged from 5;6 to 11;8 and found that even the oldest children only requested more information about half of the time. Moreover, even when the children did ask questions, their questions were often general and not specific enough to indicate what additional information was required. Ironsmith and Whitehurst suggest that several listener skills are involved in tasks of this sort: understanding the message, comparing the information given with the array of objects, formulating a query if the information is insufficient, and, for a specific query, comparing potential referents to determine the criterial attributes that distinguish them. They also suggest three levels of performance: an inability to detect ambiguity, an inability to isolate distinguishing characteristics, and an inability to perform these analyses adequately. Performance is age-related; furthermore, there is some evidence that children's performance can be improved as a result of training (Cosgrove and Patterson, 1977).

One explanation for the poor performance of children in tasks involving inadequate messages is that children do not understand that messages can be inadequate and that inadequate messages can contribute to communication failure. This view has been explored in a series of experiments in which children were asked to explain communication failure when it arises in such experimental tasks – either when they have been involved as speaker or listener, or when they act as observer (Robinson, 1981). Children aged 5 years tended to blame the listener for the failure, while children aged 7 years would more often attribute the blame to the speaker – that is, they began to locate the message as the source of the problem. Findings from other studies support the view that children cannot assess the quality of a message. For example, they will judge that the quality of the message was good if the listener makes a correct selection (Robinson and Robinson, 1977; Beal and Flavell, 1981), and they tend to confuse quantity with quality and to believe that any long message is a good one (Whitehurst, Sonnenschein and Ianfolla, 1981).

So far we have seen that, based on findings from experimental studies of referential communication, children fail to detect communicative ambiguity, and even when they do detect it, they fail to respond appropriately (see also Flavell et al., 1982). Studies of children's comprehension monitoring are related to these findings, in which it is suggested that children fail actively to monitor their own comprehension. For example, children often fail to notice inconsistencies in instructions containing glaring omissions and in stories containing blatant contradictions (Markman, 1977, 1981). As Markman suggests, comprehension is a constructive process of trying to make sense of some structured information. In order to be able to comprehend a set of instructions and to detect any inconsistencies, the child must be able mentally to enact the instructions. Similarly, comprehending a story and detecting contradiction involve using pragmatic inferences to impose a higher-order organization on the material, a process that is not necessary in the comprehension of isolated sentences. Young children appear to have difficulty in monitoring their own comprehension, because this involves a metacognitive skill over and above their ability to comprehend a message. However, if the child were able to impose structure on the instructions or story, then detecting ambiguities or inconsistencies might be easier than in the case of single ambiguous messages. The results from studies by Markman and others suggest that, in contrast with 8 year olds, children aged 6 years still have difficulty in monitoring their own comprehension due to their failure to process incoming information constructively.

Interactional aspects of clarification requests

Up until now, the way children produce and respond to clarification requests has been examined. However, it is also important to consider the role of the children's interactional partners in clarification request sequences. Two studies have been particularly interesting in this respect: one study that points to the possible interactional effects of adult input to children involved the analysis of breakdown and repair episodes in young children's (1;3–1;9) conversations with their mothers and fathers (Tomasello, Conti-Ramsden and Ewert, 1990). These investigators found that children and secondary caregiver fathers experienced more communicative breakdowns than did children and primary caregiver mothers. Furthermore, fathers requested clarification of their children more often than mothers did, and they most often used a nonspecific request (for example, "What?", "Huh?") while mothers used more specific queries (for example, "Put it where?"). Fathers also failed to acknowledge child utterances more often than mothers did. The authors interpreted these results interactionally as offering support for the Bridge Hypothesis (Gleason, 1975) which claims that fathers present children with communicative challenges that help the child prepare for communication with less familiar adults. In this sense, the breakdown and repair episodes experienced by young children with their fathers widen their experience of the three areas discussed above: awareness of possible communicative problems and solutions, awareness of the needs of different conversational partners, and awareness of the need to provide feedback and to monitor the conversational flow.

The work of Golinkoff (1986) on negotiation episodes of young children with their mothers has thrown a different light on the question: How do interactional features affect the child's pragmatic and conversational development? Golinkoff carried out a longitudinal study of how preverbal infants aged 1;0–1;7 managed to communicate with their mothers. She found that infants' communicative attempts were often unsuccessful (around 50 percent of the time) but after failure, infants and mothers worked together to establish the infant's intent. This working together had a structure which Golinkoff refers to as *negotiation episodes*. Negotiation episodes have four components: the infant's initial signal, the mother's comprehension failure, infant repairs, and episode outcome. For example:

Baby:	(Looks and reaches in direction of food and table.) *Initial signal*.
Mother:	(Mother looks at food.) What do you want? (Looks at baby.)

Comprehension failure.
Baby:	(Baby holds original signal.)

Repair or repetition.
Mother:	(Looks at baby and offers food.) This?

Reformulation.
Baby:	(Looks at mother and accepts food.)

Outcome: success.

These negotiation episodes are contrasted with episodes referred to as *immediate successes* in which the mother readily understands the intent of the infant's signal and *missed attempts* in which the mother fails to pick up on the infant's signal. Interestingly, negotiation episodes have an average length of 7.3 turns which is in line with the case-study presented by Wells (1981) that mother–infant interactions are anything but brief, but often involve a number of turns that focus on a single topic and involve negotiation of meaning. From participation in negotiation episodes, Golinkoff argues, infants appear to learn about pragmatics and communication. First, infants may learn how to establish shared reference. We have seen how preverbal infants take increasing responsibility for initiating interaction and sharing reference. As time goes on, infants recognize that the listener must have the same visual experience as him- or herself in order to establish joint reference. Negotiation episodes provide an opportunity for the child to practice further the strategies necessary to establish a discourse topic. Recall that negotiation episodes in Golinkoff's work only included those episodes initiated by the child, so that the burden for establishing shared reference rested on the infant. Secondly, negotiation episodes may help the child learn Grice's (1975) cooperative principle for communication. This important principle directs the speaker to signal clearly, to monitor the listener's comprehension, and to signal to the listener whether his or her interpretation of the interactive contribution is indeed correct. Finally, negotiation episodes may help the child focus on communication problems and learn possible solutions such as repair.

Children's self-repairs

This section is concluded with a look at children's self-repairs in their spontaneous speech. Self-repairs occur when a speaker corrects his or her own utterance and thus involves a process of monitoring the utterance in order to prevent potential communication breakdown (Evans, 1985). They can take the form of filled and unfilled pauses, repetitions, corrections, and abandoned utterances. Self-repairs may have various causes: planning errors involving word-finding problems; execution errors such as phonological reversals; and interactional problems, such as identifying referents sufficiently for a listener.

Clark and Andersen (1979) have distinguished between two types of self-repair: repairs to the linguistic system, for example, grammatical self-corrections, and repairs for the listener, which are motivated by the need to be understood. Repairs to the linguistic system provide useful information about children's developing language skill (see McTear, 1985a, pp.188 *et seq.* for discussion and examples). Repairs for the listener are interesting in terms of children developing pragmatic skills because they illustrate children's attempts to adapt their message to their perceptions of their listener's needs. For example, in the following examples the children substitute noun phrases for pronouns and thus make their utterance more explicit for the listener:

H: And she's (1.1) this little girl's two year old
S: She. My friend Heather knows how to take it off herself

In summary, the study of communication breakdown and repair in conversations involving young children provides important information about the children's developing pragmatic competence. Children show an ability from an early age to respond to requests for clarification when their utterances have been unclear or misunderstood. They are also able to make requests for clarification in naturally occurring conversational contexts when they have failed to understand the utterances of their conversational partner. However, when higher and more abstract levels of performance are involved, as indicated in studies of children's judgments of message quality in referential communication tasks as well as their comprehension monitoring under experimental conditions, it has been found that children are still deficient in the ability to detect and repair communication breakdown until early adolescence. Finally, studies of children's self-repairs in spontaneous conversation provide some insight into their ability to monitor their own speech and to make adjustments for their listener. Thus the study of communication breakdown and repair provides a wide range of information on children's pragmatic skills.

Difficulties with clarification requests

There are many occasions when conversation may break down as a result of an unclear utterance or a misunderstanding on the part of the listener. It should be expected that breakdowns might occur more frequently in the case of language-impaired children because their utterances are less likely to be understood. The ability to repair conversational breakdowns requires a listener to recognize when an utterance has not been understood and to request appropriate clarification, while a speaker has to respond to the request of a listener with the required clarification. Making and responding to clarification requests depends on linguistic skills enabling children to revise previous utterances or monitor their comprehension, as well as on pragmatic knowledge of the obligations of conversational participants to clarify actual or potential misunderstandings.

It has generally been found that language-impaired children recognize that clarification requests require a response (Gallagher and Darnton, 1978; Pearl, Donahue and Bryan, 1983; Porter and Conti-Ramsden, 1987). What these studies suggest is that language-impaired children can fulfil the pragmatic demands of clarification requests in spite of linguistic deficiencies. For example, in a case study of a child recorded in mother–child interaction between the ages of 4;6 and 5;3, the child, in spite of limited phonologic and syntactic abilities, usually responded to his mother's clarification requests so that most clarification episodes terminated satisfactorily, while the instances of communication breakdown in every case appeared to represent the child's unwillingness to clarify rather than his inability (Porter and Conti-Ramsden, 1987).

However, the responses produced by language-impaired children have often been found to be less sophisticated and more inappropriate responses than those of their language- and age-matched peers. Gallagher and Darnton (1978) found that the responses of their subjects were less elaborate than would be predicted by their acquired level of grammatical ability. Similarly, while Pearl, Donahue and Bryan (1983) reported that in a descriptive task both language-learning-disabled children and nondisabled children were able to respond to explicit as well as implicit requests for clarification, in a task demanding more elaborate use of language it was found that the descriptions of the language-learning-disabled children were syntactically less complex than those of their age-matched peers (Donahue, Pearl and Bryan, 1982). The child studied by Porter and Conti-Ramsden (1987) also used a basic strategy of repeating his previous response rather than revising its linguistic form in sequences in which the mother repeated her nonspecific request for clarification. In each case the responses of the language-impaired children are qualitatively different from those of normal language-learning children who, regardless of language stage, revised the linguistic form of their original utterance when confronted with a neutral request and tended to develop more sophisticated revision strategies as their language developed (Gallagher, 1977).

These differences would seem to indicate a relationship between linguistic abilities and revision strategies. Such a relationship is to be expected, because more sophisticated revision strategies require more complex linguistic structures. However, there are reasons to look beyond level of linguistic development as the only explanation of the less elaborate responses of language-impaired children. Recall that in the Gallagher and Darnton (1978) study the level of the revisions of the language-impaired group was even lower than would be expected from their language stage and did not seem to develop in keeping with developments in the children's language. Furthermore, recent studies comparing the responses by linguistically normal and language-impaired children to sequences of clarification requests have suggested that, in addition to a linguistic deficiency, the language-impaired children showed less awareness of their listener's needs, because their inappropriate responses did not accommodate the listener's needs in any way (Brinton, et al., 1986; Brinton, Fujiki and Sonnenberg, 1988). The language-impaired group appeared to be more adversely affected as the complexity of the task increased. Finally, they may also have interpreted the repeated clarification requests as a value judgment on their responses and may have discontinued the sequence rather than risk producing what they believed would be another incorrect response. In other words, the children did not lack repair strategies but rather lacked persistence in applying them.

As far as the production of clarification requests by language-impaired children is concerned, there is evidence of a lack of awareness of the need to request clarification as well as a qualitative difference in the requests made. Brinton and Fujiki (1982) found that their language-impaired subjects produced fewer clarification requests than their normal-speaking peers, while Donahue, Pearl and Bryan (1980) reported that, in a referential communication task involving listening to a message and then selecting the correct object described in the message and in which subjects were presented with informative as well as ambiguous messages, the language-learning-disabled children as well as younger children were less likely to request clarification than their comparison groups of ambiguous messages. The requests of language-impaired children also appear to be less sophisticated and to take the form mainly of nonspecific requests for repetition (Hargrove, Straka and Medders, 1988), although a developmental trend towards more sophisticated requests was reported in the case study of Porter and Conti-Ramsden (1987).

In attempting to explain the nature of language-impaired children's clarification requests, it is necessary to distinguish carefully between linguistic and other factors. It is possible to evoke linguistic impairment as an explanation for the less elaborate clarification requests produced by language-impaired children, because the ability to produce more elaborate requests depends on knowledge of the appropriate linguistic structures. The production of fewer requests could also be related to linguistic deficiencies – either a failure to notice that an utterance has not been understood, i.e. deficient comprehension monitoring, or an inability to produce the appropriate clarification request. However, there are reasons to suspect that there are other causes that are only indirectly related to linguistic problems. The study by Donahue, Pearl and Bryan (1980), mentioned earlier, was designed to assess the contribution of linguistic knowledge to children's ability to request clarification of ambiguous messages when playing the listener role. As shown, language-learning-disabled children produced fewer clarification requests of partially informative and uninformative messages. However, their problems were not due to an inability to recognize inadequate messages, because in a second task they were able to assess the adequacy of the messages by predicting whether an imaginary listener would be able to understand them and select the correct referent. Furthermore, an analysis of the requests that they did produce indicated that they had the linguistic abilities to produce appropriate clarification requests. One possibility is that the children did not understand the conversational rule that listeners are obliged to initiate the repair of conversational breakdown. Another possibility is that, as a result of a history of communicative failures, they may have been led to believe that failure to understand a message was due to their own deficient comprehension, especially if they also believed that their adult partners were unlikely to produce inadequate messages. In other words, the children appeared to be placing an over-reliance on the Gricean maxim of quantity which requires that cooperative speakers should provide informative messages but not include more details than are necessary. An analysis of the children's picture selection strategies supports this hypothesis, because the children tended to select the picture with the fewest features, apparently under the assumption that the adult would have specified the additional details if other referents had been intended. Similar findings, as well as children's explicit justifications of their responses to ambiguous messages, have been reported for normally developing children, as discussed earlier (see studies by Sonnenschein and Whitehurst, 1980; Jackson and Jacobs, 1982; Bredart, 1984). Thus ironically the observation of one of the maxims of cooperative conversation leads to an apparent conversational disability.

Presupposition

In Chapter 2 it was shown how the term "presupposition" has been used in a wide range of ways to refer generally to assumptions that speakers make when they utter a sentence. A more precise use of the term was introduced within pragmatics to refer to assumptions that are built into linguistic expressions. To recap, there are some verbs that trigger presuppositions. For example:

John managed to stop in time
(presupposes) John tried to stop in time

John realized that he had failed the exam
(presupposes) John failed the exam

Most developmental work involving this more precise view of presupposition has been concerned with children's ability to make judgments about the assumptions triggered by mental verbs such as *know, forget, remember, think* and *believe*. The first three of these verbs have been called *factive* verbs (Kiparsky and Kiparsky, 1970). What this means is that a speaker using these verbs in the main clause of an utterance is assuming the truth of the complement clause. For example, in uttering

William forgot that he had bought some rice

a speaker is committed to the truth of *William bought some rice*. This presupposition also holds under negation, so that

William didn't forget that he had bought some rice

also presupposes *William bought some rice*. However, nonfactive verbs such as *think* and *believe* do not give rise to these presuppositions. For example:

Alan thought that he had bought some rice

does not commit the speaker to the truth of the proposition *Alan bought some rice*.

Studies of children's understanding of the assumptions which may or may not be triggered by mental verbs such as these have typically involved the children in making judgments about the truth value of isolated sentences. Abbeduto and Rosenberg (1985) presented children with sentences such as

Sharon remembered that Clive stole a radio

The children had to judge the truth of the sentence "Did Clive steal a radio?" by answering "Yes", "No", or "Don't know". (The answer *don't know* would be appropriate in the case of nonfactive verbs such as *think*.)

Results from these studies have been inconsistent, suggesting methodological problems (Milford, 1989). Abbeduto and Rosenberg (1985) found that children have acquired the presuppositions of mental verbs by age 4, while others, such as Scoville and Gordon (1980) claim that children are still acquiring aspects of this ability at age 14. One factor is the method of assessment used in the studies. For example, assessments of the truth values of isolated sentences may be biased by particular response strategies, such as an unwillingness to use the *don't know* response because it could imply ignorance, or by a tendency to ignore the main verb and attend only to the verb in the complement clause (Hopmann and Maratsos, 1978). A second factor is the difference between the particular verbs used in the studies. While some verbs such as *know* and *think* seem to be less complex regarding whether they trigger presuppositions or not, others, such as *remember* and *believe*, appear to be more difficult. Moreover, judgments appear to differ according to whether the verbs are used in positive as opposed to negative sentences. Thus it appears that knowledge of presuppositions triggered by mental verbs has to be learned on an item-by-item basis and is affected by the semantic complexity of the verb in question (Hopmann and Maratsos, 1978).

Milford (1989) designed a study that took into account these methodological difficulties. The ability to understand the presuppositions triggered by mental verbs was assessed in a story context in which subjects heard a short story and were then asked questions about the story. The following is an example of one of the stories used (Milford, 1989, p. 137):

One morning, they were all sitting at the table in the kitchen. Daddy was reading the paper. The children were all playing with a jigsaw. One of the children knocked the jigsaw off the table and it fell on to the floor. That night, Mum asked about the jigsaw.

Mark said that he picked up the pieces of the jigsaw. Sarah forgot that she had knocked the jigsaw off the table. Kathryn thought that she had knocked the jigsaw off the table.

Questions
1. Who knocked the jigsaw off the table?
2. Where were the children playing?
3. Who was reading the paper?

As can be seen, questions 2 and 3 involve information that is stated explicitly in the story, while question 1 can only be answered correctly if the subject understands the differences between the verbs *forget* and *think* in terms of whether they trigger a presupposition. Subjects of the experiments were children aged 4, 7 and 10, as well as adults. There were 12 verb pairings, involving the factive verbs *know*, *forget* and *remember*, each paired with the nonfactive verbs *think* and *believe*, in affirmative and negative sentence conditions. The results supported the view that presupposition is acquired over a long period of time and is related to the complexity of individual mental verbs. For example, scores for the pairing *think/forget* were 50 percent at age 4, increasing gradually to 100 percent for adults, while for the pairing *believe/forget*, 4 and 7 year olds scored 10 percent, 10 year olds scored 40 percent, and adults 100 percent.

Although there have been few studies of presupposition in children, it is clear that the ability to make the correct inferences depending on which mental verb is used is important for a child's ability to understand stories and similar examples of continuous discourse, and to be able to assume information that is not stated explicitly in the text. Milford (1989) reviewed reading material for 7 year olds and found that a wide variety of presuppositional triggers were used. If, as the studies of Milford and others suggest, children still have difficulty with presupposition into early adolescence, then it is likely that they will not be able to understand fully such reading material.

Presuppositions associated with mental verbs are closely related to investigations of children's developing theory of mind (discussed in more detail in Chapter 6), which is concerned with the ability to infer mental states from observable events and to use these inferred states to make predictions about behavior. In studies of presupposition the child has to process information involving mental states and has to make the correct assumptions about the truth of information that is not stated explicitly. Some of the more advanced studies of children's theory of mind require this ability to make presuppositions, as shown presently, so that there is a close relationship between this specific pragmatic ability and children's sociocognitive abilities.

Making inferences

In Chapter 2 several different uses of the term "inference" were discussed. Deductive (or logical) inferences refer to valid conclusions which can be derived from a set of premises. Pragmatic inferences are assumptions of what a speaker means which go beyond what was actually said. In other words, pragmatic inferences involve reading into an utterance meanings in addition to its literal meaning. Related to pragmatic inferences are bridging inferences, which enable a listener to make sense of a series of sentences in a text by inferring connections that were not actually made explicit in the text.

Pragmatic inferences involve the integration of incoming information into existing structures or frameworks of knowledge and experience. For example, to understand relationships between events in a story, it is necessary to be able to relate the events in terms of temporal and causal relationships. Children's ability to make these sorts of inferences have been investigated in several studies. Children have been shown to use their prior experience and expectations when inferring information from natural oral discourse (Hildyard, 1979). They are able to infer relationships among propositions as represented by pictures (Paris and Mahoney, 1974) and they can complete missing links to order a set of pictures by using their knowledge of causal and temporal relationships between events (Brown and Murphy, 1975; Brown and Hurtig, 1983).

One missing element from studies of children's inferential abilities is an examination of the knowledge structures that enable children to make these inferences. In fact, it is doubtful whether it is possible to separate the ability to derive conversational implicatures and to make pragmatic inferences from cognitive issues involving knowledge structures, particularly when the implicatures and inferences depend on the ability of the listener to work out what is meant on the basis of general world knowledge as well as what knowledge is assumed to be shared with the speaker. There is a review of some work that sheds light on these issues in the examination of cognitive aspects of language use in Chapter 6.

Concluding remarks

In this chapter the development of pragmatic ability in children has been reviewed in detail and the sorts of problems that some children experience when using language in everyday communication have been examined. On the basis of this review it should be possible for clinicians and researchers to appreciate the different aspects of language use that may cause children difficulty and to consider these aspects in their assessment and treatment procedures.

Following this descriptive account it is necessary to look at ways of explaining pragmatic disability. Two questions are particularly relevant in this respect:

1. Are there different types of pragmatic disability?
2. How does a child's pragmatic ability relate to other abilities and disabilities?

It seems reasonable to assume that there could be different types of pragmatic disability. It is generally agreed that communication involves the integration of linguistic, cognitive, and social skills (Shatz, 1983b; Johnston, 1985). Thus a child could be competent in one skill relevant to communication but deficient in others, or, alternatively, a child could be competent in each of the relevant skills but unable to integrate them appropriately to serve the demands of communication.

In order to answer these questions relationships between pragmatic ability/disability and other skills are considered. In the next chapter the relationship between linguistic and pragmatic development is examined, while in Chapter 6 alternative explanations are investigated in terms of cognitive, sociocognitive, and affective–emotional factors; in addition, it is shown how some aspects of language use are closely related to language ability while others are dependent on other factors – in other words, that there are different types of pragmatic disability.

Chapter 5
Explaining Pragmatic Disability: Linguistic and Pragmatic Factors

The view that linguistic ability determines the development of pragmatic skills underlies most work on pragmatic disability in children. It seems intuitively obvious that some knowledge of linguistic structures is necessary for communicative tasks involving language – such as making requests, producing narratives, or using referring expressions to describe objects or persons. However, few studies have explicitly attempted to relate children's linguistic abilities to their pragmatic abilities in order to determine causal relationships. In this chapter, potential relationships are indicated and some relevant studies reviewed. At the same time those aspects of pragmatic ability are considered which seem to be independent of language ability. Following this, a more detailed examination is made of the assumptions underlying group design studies of the pragmatic disabilities of language-impaired children, because it is in these studies that potential relationships between linguistic and pragmatic disability have been most explicitly addressed. In conclusion the other side of the coin is examined – the role that pragmatic factors play in the development of linguistic ability.

The effects of linguistic ability on the development of pragmatic skills

In this section the different aspects of pragmatic development discussed in the previous chapter are examined and the relationship of the acquisition of these pragmatic skills to a child's linguistic development is explored. An examination is made of more subtle ways in which linguistic impairment can affect children's communicative performance and of some alternative explanations.

Turn-taking

Turn-taking is a primary aspect of conversation. Efficient turn-taking depends on precise timing so as to avoid situations in which more than one speaker talks at the same time or where lengthy gaps occur between turns. Furthermore, turn-taking requires listeners to monitor the current turn closely and to predict when the speaker might be about to stop, so that the next turn can start without delay and without causing overlap. Note that conversational turn-taking is more advanced than turn-taking in proto-conversations, where caregiver and child simply alternate behaviors without any need to predict turn-completion points. Any semblance of timing is imposed by careful coordination on the part of the caregiver. In conversational turn-taking, however, the listener has to bring to bear a knowledge of syntactic structure as well as an understanding of prosodic cues in order to determine whether the turn is nearing potential completion.

Children's linguistic deficiencies may have an adverse effect on their ability to take turns effectively in conversation, because turn-taking involves the ability of a child to integrate pragmatic and linguistic knowledge. It was seen how, in the study of the turn-taking abilities of language-impaired children by Craig and Evans (1989), the children were competent in the pragmatic aspects of turn-taking but had difficulties in those aspects that required specific linguistic abilities, in particular the skills involved in encoding and decoding sufficiently rapidly for precision-timed turn-taking.

However, there are some aspects of turn-taking that seem to be independent of linguistic ability. The ability to assign and take turns in conversation evolves out of reciprocal interactions between caregivers and young infants in the prelinguistic stage. Indeed, as seen from the discussion of communication in early infancy, children are able to engage in reciprocal behaviors involving turn-taking before they have acquired any language at all. Thus knowledge of where it is appropriate to take turns in conversation, and knowledge of the rules for turn allocation in dialogue as well as in multi-party talk, would seem to draw on pragmatic ability – that is, the ability to relate the use of language to its context of use. This applies for a variety of different social contexts, involving symmetrical as well as nonsymmetrical relationships between the speakers.

Language-impaired children do not appear to have difficulties in turn allocation itself. For example, Kysela et al.(1990) found that language-impaired children at the one-word stage compared favorably with their normally developing peers in their ability to take turns in conversation. Similar findings for older children are reported by Craig and Evans (1989) as far as sentence-initial overlaps were concerned – that is, there were few cases in which adults and children attempted to start talking at the same time and any cases of simultaneous speech arising from such turn exchange errors were usually repaired by the child giving up the floor. Thus, as far as language-impaired children are concerned, turn allocation does not appear to be problematic, although predicting possible turn completions, which depends on linguistic skills of encoding and decoding, is problematic for these children, as shown earlier. However, it has been reported that other groups of children, in particular autistic children, have specific problems with appropriate turn-taking (Fay and Schuler, 1980). Baltaxe (1977) found that autistic children had difficulty in moving between speaker and hearer roles in conversation, with the result that they may remain in the speaker role for too long (Bernard-Opitz, 1982) or in the hearer role for too long (McCaleb and Prizant, 1985). Autistic children also fail to use eye contact to signal turn-taking (Mirenda, Donnellan and Yoder, 1983). Thus autistic children appear to have a specific difficulty with turn-taking which is independent of their language abilities, although this impairment may be related either to affective/emotional problems (Hobson, 1986a,b) or to a sociocognitive deficiency in assessing the mental states of other people (Baron-Cohen, 1988). These alternative explanations are discussed in Chapter 6.

Initiations

Initiating conversational exchanges would seem to require some degree of linguistic ability. Being able to refer to persons or objects not present in the immediate environment has to be achieved linguistically – for example, by the use of a relative clause (e.g. "The man who was speaking to you last night" in which the relative clause *who was speaking to you last night* helps to identify the person in question). Tense marking in the verb may also be relevant, as in the distinction between *the toys I play with* as opposed to *the toys I played with*. Highlighting the main informational content of a message requires the ability to distinguish between old and new information in relation to the conversation so far – for example, knowing that a phrase such as *the boy* is normally used to refer back to someone previously mentioned, whereas *a boy* is used on first mention. For the listener, the problem is in reverse – recognizing the significance of these linguistic cues for the interpretation of the discourse. Knowing the need for these distinctions is one part of the problem; however, being able to make the distinctions depends on the child having previously acquired the relevant linguistic items.

There are, however, some aspects of conversational initiations that appear to be more or less independent of linguistic ability. Getting the listener's attention requires a command of attention-getting devices, some of which are linguistic and some of which are nonlinguistic, as well as the knowledge of which device is more appropriate to use on a particular occasion. Similarly, the use of appropriate attention-directing devices involves not only linguistic knowledge of the particular structures involved, but also the ability to judge which linguistic or nonlinguistic form is appropriate in the context; this includes the situation of utterance as well as inferences involving the listener's current state of knowledge. It is also clear that this ability is distinct from linguistic ability because infants are able to direct the attention of their caregivers to objects around them before they have acquired language.

Pragmatic ability is also involved in the more complex attention-directing tasks assessed in referential communication experiments, in which children are required to describe a picture so that it can be identified by a listener from a set of similar pictures differing in perhaps only one aspect. While the ability to describe the pictures at all requires linguistic knowledge, the ability to determine which information can be included as necessary and which can be omitted as redundant requires an assessment of the information relative to the context – that is, the information contained in the other pictures as well as the knowledge state of the listener.

Autistic children seem to be deficient in the use of appropriate attention-getting devices such as establishing eye contact or using the listener's name (Fay and Schuler, 1980). As far as attention-directing is concerned, children with learning difficulties appear to be deficient in providing information which would help their listener to identify the referents of their messages beyond what would be predicted by their linguistic and cognitive abilities (King, 1989), while autistic children have difficulties with distinguishing between old and new information (Baltaxe, 1977) and tend to initiate inappropriately by asking the same question over and over again (Hurtig, Ensrud and Tomblin, 1982). There are several possible explanations for these difficulties. The children may fail to appreciate the conversational principles involved in initiating conversation, such as the need to get the listener's attention, to specify adequately the objects referred to in the message, or to assess the appropriacy of a question. However, a child who is aware of these principles may still have difficulties in applying them appropriately because of a failure to assess the listener's needs – whether the listener is already attending, can identify the objects being referred to, or has understood information that has been conveyed. An inability to assess the listener's needs rather than to be aware of which pragmatic devices to use is a consequence of sociocognitive difficulties, which will be examined in Chapter 6.

Speech acts

Speech acts are often cited as a prime example of pragmatic ability. Speech acts are concerned with the functions rather than the forms of language. On the one hand, as stressed previously, the ability to use and understand speech acts depends on both linguistic and pragmatic skills. For example, making polite requests depends on the prior acquisition of verb forms such as *could* and *would* as well as complex grammatical structures such as *would you mind* + *verb* + *-ing* (e.g. "Would you mind shutting the door"). It also depends on the ability to distinguish between the literal meaning of an utterance and its indirectly conveyed meaning – mainly a question of linguistic competence. On the other hand, the ability to understand the conditions under which particular linguistic forms can fulfil particular communicative functions related to particular contexts of use is mainly a question of pragmatic competence.

It has been frequently reported that language-impaired children may use a restricted range of speech acts. For example, they fail to use language to describe and inform spontaneously; instead they use language mainly to direct the listener's attention. In other cases language-impaired children are nonassertive in conversation and their contributions are limited to back-channel responses (i.e. verbal and nonverbal devices such as *umbmm* and nodding which indicate attention without taking the conversational initiative). One reason for this nonassertiveness may be that the child has linguistic deficiencies that make responding in conversation and maintaining an ongoing topic or introducing a new topic problematic (Rosinski-McClendon and Newhoff, 1987). Certainly, if the child's range of speech acts is inferior to that of age-matched peers but equals that of language-matched peers, then there is reasonable support for attributing the problems to linguistic deficiencies.

The adoption of a passive role in conversation could be a consequence of poor comprehension skills, because an inability to understand the messages of their partners would make conversational participation difficult for these children. To test this hypothesis it would be necessary to test the children's comprehension skills. Comprehension also affects a child's ability to recognize and respond to indirect speech acts. It has been reported that language-impaired children, and autistic children in particular, have difficulty with the comprehension of indirect speech acts and tend to respond to the literal rather than indirect meanings. Thus being able to decide whether an utterance such as "Can you put the ball into the truck" is a question or a request may depend on the extent to which the child can use prior context (see, for example, Shatz, Bernstein and Shulman, 1980), or can combine evidence from the current situation as well as an assessment of the speaker's probable intentions.

The fact that some children adopt a mainly nonresponsive or a nonassertive role in conversation may be due to various factors other than linguistic ability. Children may be unaware of the social obligation to be responsive in conversation. Nonresponsiveness may also be due to personality factors, as in the case of an extremely shy or withdrawn child. Alternatively, this unwillingness may be the result of previous communication failures which have convinced the child that defensive strategies in conversation will decrease the likelihood of further such failures (Bryan, 1986; Donahue, 1987). Indeed, the cause of the difficulty could involve a combination of these factors.

An alternative explanation, in terms of interactional factors, is suggested by a study of adult–child interaction which showed that the mothers of language-impaired children with normal comprehension initiated dialogue significantly more often than mothers of nonlanguage-impaired children, while the language-impaired children initiated dialogue significantly less often than the nonlanguage-impaired children (Conti-Ramsden, 1990). The mothers of the language-impaired children used more questions and directives, thus forcing their children into a more passive role, possibly in an effort to engage the child more effectively in dialogue and to maintain the interaction. Conversely, the mothers of the nonlanguage-impaired children tended to use semantically related utterances such as recasts and other contingent replies which are less regulative discourse devices. Thus the passive role adopted by the language-impaired child can be explained in terms of interactional factors, such as different maternal strategies which are in turn a response to the children's speech characteristics, such as restricted intelligibility on the part of the language-impaired children.

Finally, there are socioaffective explanations, particularly in the case of autistic children, who are often reported as being nonassertive in conversation. In this case the explanation lies not in their linguistic ability so much as in a lack of the required sociability. So the same symptoms can have different origins and the relationship between the observable behavior and its explanation can only be determined by obtaining relevant supporting data, whether these are scores of comprehension or sociability ratings, or by careful analysis of the interactional context and the respective contributions of the conversational participants.

As far as pragmatic aspects of speech acts are concerned, we have seen how the use of speech acts involves an appreciation of appropriacy conditions – whether it is appropriate, for example, to make a request on this occasion to this person – that are quite distinct from considerations of the linguistic forms of the speech acts. The fact that children use primitive forms of speech acts before they acquire language again indicates that this aspect of communicative competence is independent of linguistic ability.

Autistic children often violate conversational principles of acceptability and politeness (Baltaxe, 1977). Similarly, language-learning-disabled children have difficulty in making adjustments in conversational style to suit the characteristics of their listeners or the nature of the task in hand (Donahue, 1981). However, it is important to examine the causes of these deficiencies carefully. To use a speech act appropriately a child must have

- the linguistic resources
- the ability to discriminate between listener and situational features
- an appreciation of how to vary speech according to these features.

In other words, when a child has difficulties with speech acts it is necessary to consider whether the difficulties are explained in terms of one or more of these aspects, because the causes of the difficulties may vary from child to child.

Clarification requests

Clarification sequences involve a combination of linguistic and pragmatic knowledge. Clarification requests occur when a listener realizes that an utterance is unclear. This involves the linguistic ability to process utterances and the pragmatic ability to interpret them relative to the current context. Responding to requests for clarification can involve more than just repeating the problematic utterance – in many cases, it is necessary to paraphrase in some way. This can involve reordering sentence constituents, changing sentence mood (e.g. from imperative to interrogative), as well as the use of ellipsis in order to avoid repeating parts of the utterance that are judged to have been understood.

Linguistic impairment can affect a child's ability to make appropriate conversational adjustments and revisions. Modifying syntactic constructions to take account of different types of listener or to express various degrees of indirectness may place undue demands on the linguistic resources of language-impaired children (Fey and Leonard, 1983). Similarly, the ability to revise utterances in response to clarification requests by using paraphrases or lexical substitutions is restricted for children with limited linguistic knowledge (Gallagher and Darnton, 1978; Brinton et al.,1986; Brinton, Fujiki and Sonnenberg, 1988). However, as far as adjustments to the listener are concerned, there is the alternative explanation of an inability to assess the listener's needs. In this case the problem is sociocognitive. To rule out this possibility it would be necessary to have independent evidence that the child's sociocognitive skills were unimpaired.

Understanding the obligations of speakers and listeners to keep conversation flowing smoothly and to repair misunderstanding is a basic conversational skill. As shown in Chapter 4, language-impaired children appear to be aware of the obligation to respond to and make clarification requests, although the level of sophistication of their requests and responses is determined by their linguistic abilities and they seem less aware of the needs of their listeners (Brinton et al., 1986; Brinton, Fujiki and Sonnenberg, 1988).

However, some children appear to be deficient in the production of clarification requests even when they have the necessary linguistic skills. For example, in experimental studies children have failed to request clarification of ambiguous or unclear messages, even in situations where they would be unable to select the correct object (Donahue, Pearl and

Bryan, 1980). Several explanations are possible. Perhaps the children failed to notice that the messages were inadequate. However, this explanation was ruled out in one study in which the children demonstrated in a follow-up task that they could in fact recognize message inadequacy (Donahue, Pearl and Bryan, 1980). One possibility is that the children avoided clarification requests because they did not wish to draw attention to their inability to understand – possibly as a result of previous experiences of communication failure. It is also possible that children assume that adults will always produce adequate messages and that any problems are a consequence of their own deficient skills of comprehension. In other words, children may place an over-reliance on conversational maxims, such as the Gricean maxim of quantity, under which it is assumed that a speaker only says as much as is required (and no more). These children need to learn when normal conversational principles are being flouted or disregarded for a particular communicative purpose – such as, in this case, an experimental set-up.

Other ways in which linguistic impairments affect pragmatic ability

A description has already been given of some of the ways in which linguistic impairments can affect a child's ability to use language to achieve particular communicative goals. In this section some less obvious examples are presented of the effects of linguistic deficiencies on children's pragmatic ability.

Many children who are described as having pragmatic disability are reported as having problems in word-finding and the expression of temporal and causal relationships. These problems affect their ability to use language effectively.

As far as word-finding problems are concerned, children may have difficulty in targeting the required words. In some cases, as shown in a wide range of naming tasks, this seems to be a result of not being able to access known words sufficiently rapidly (German, 1979). This disability often leads to the adoption of compensatory strategies, such as circumlocution, or the use of imprecise words and other indications of word-finding difficulty such as hesitations and false starts (Wiig and Semel, 1984). The effects on social interaction of such word-finding problems can be serious. For example, Silliman (1984) reports that the classmates of language-learning-disabled children who had such word-finding problems found great difficulty in attending to the narratives of the learning-disabled children on account of the numerous dysfluencies. Similar social consequences could be expected in other contexts.

Children may also have difficulties due to unusual or over-restricted use of lexical items, such as spatial prepositions (Smedley, 1989). The problems may be due to "rigid concept boundaries". For example, a child saying "The clock is by the wall" may believe that *on* is to be used only to refer to locations on the horizontal plane. More generally, children may restrict their use of words to their most obvious, literal meanings with a resultant limitation on their expressive language or in their ability to understand metaphorical and less literal meanings of words.

Deficiencies in language for expressing temporal and causal relations will affect children's ability to order events in a narrative and perceive relationships between events involving consequence or motivation. Children may have difficulty in understanding and responding appropriately to *when, how* and *why* questions, or they may use *because* to mean *and* or *so* (for example: "It is six o'clock because Mike is getting up"). Smedley (1989) found children with these difficulties whose nonverbal cognitive processes were not impaired, which suggests that their problems were linguistic, with consequences for their ability to produce and comprehend extended discourse. Similar difficulties with the use of spatial, temporal and causal relations are reported in the case study of McTear (1985b).

Language-impaired children have particular difficulties with certain aspects of syntax and tend to omit determiners, auxiliaries and sentence subjects in contexts where these are obligatory (Fletcher and Garman, 1988). Omission of determiners means that the child will not be able to mark the distinction between old and new information which enables listeners to follow the connections in a piece of discourse. A lack of auxiliaries means that the child is unable to express certain meanings conveyed by auxiliary verbs, such as degree of possibility, while omission of the sentence subject makes it difficult for the listener to retrieve the referent of the omitted subject. As with other examples, it is more problematic if we wish to explain these omissions. A failure to use determiners could be a result of the child not yet being aware of a need to distinguish between old and new information, while omission of sentence subjects may be due to the child's assumption that, if the referent of the sentence subject is mutually available to speaker and listener, then there is no need to specify it. Thus syntactic immaturity may give rise to pragmatic deficiencies, although equally the child's syntactic deficiencies may be attributable to pragmatic factors.

Group design studies revisitied

In Chapter 3 group design studies were considered as one way in which to investigate pragmatic disability. However, group design studies are also useful for investigating the relationship between linguistic ability and pragmatic skills. The basic assumption in these studies is that children who are language-impaired will also be deficient in their use of language. In other words, their use of language is closely related to their level of linguistic ability and any deficiencies in language structure will affect their ability to use language. Thus the usual prediction in these studies is that language-impaired children will be similar in their level of pragmatic development to children younger than themselves who are at the same language level as themselves.

There are, however, four possible outcomes of such group design studies and it is worth examining each of these in some detail in order to explore the relationship between linguistic and pragmatic abilities. Each of these possible outcomes is discussed in turn and relevant research findings presented.

1. The pragmatic skills of the language-impaired group match those of their language-matched peers (and are inferior to those of their age-matched peers)

This is the expected finding of group design studies of pragmatic disability, because it supports the hypothesis that children who are language-impaired will have difficulties in using language to communicate. Many studies have, in fact, confirmed this hypothesis. However, as will be seen, even in these cases the assumed relationships between language and language use may not be as clear cut as would first appear.

Children with specific language impairments have been found to be similar to younger normally developing children matched for language level in several aspects of communication – turn-taking ability at the one-word stage (Kysela et al., 1990); range of different speech acts used (Rom and Bliss, 1981; Leonard et al., 1982); their ability to adjust their speech to their listener's characteristics (Leonard, 1983); the level of sophistication of their responses to requests for clarification (Gallagher and Darnton, 1978; Hargrove, Straka and Medders, 1988); and the level of focus and substitution devices used to continue ongoing discourse (van Kleeck and Frankel, 1981). In each case their choice and range of linguistic features were constrained by their grammatical immaturity. Similarly, Prinz and Ferrier (1983) found that children's language levels – as measured by scores on a sentence repetition task – were correlated with the range of request forms that they produced and the levels of politeness that they perceived. These results are as expected. If children have difficulty with particular grammatical forms such as auxiliaries, which are also used to construct polite requests, then we might expect that their grammatical and pragmatic skills would be closely related.

Another area in which grammatical ability may affect pragmatic performance is in the production of informative messages. Feagans and Short (1984) found that children's oral language deficits co-occurred with difficulties in producing narratives, due to lack of syntactic structures and

124   Pragmatic Disability in Children

vocabulary inflexibility. Syntactic difficulties also appeared to affect the children's ability to paraphrase in their responses to clarification requests, while limited vocabulary – as well as word-retrieval problems – affected the ability of language-impaired children to introduce new referents explicitly to their listeners (Liles, 1985a,b).

Some studies, while finding that language-disabled children performed similarly to their language-matched peers for some aspects of communication, also reported that their performance was worse than predicted for other aspects. For example, in a study of conversational responsiveness and assertiveness, in which language-impaired children with ages ranging from 4;1 to 5;9 were matched by MLU (mean length of utterance) with language-normal children, it was found that the language-impaired children were similar to their language-matched peers in terms of conversational assertiveness, as measured by the extent to which they would continue a topic following no response from their listener or would attempt to maintain their topic following a topic change initiated by their adult partner (Rosinski-McClendon and Newhoff, 1987). In the case of topic continuations following no response by the investigator, both groups tended to assert themselves verbally with similar frequency. Both groups were minimally assertive in the face of a topic change introduced by the adult investigator and tended simply to follow the adult's lead. However, when conversational responsiveness was assessed, as measured by frequency and topical relevance of responses to questions inserted as on-topic probes during a free conversation with an adult, the language-impaired group demonstrated a lower level of responsiveness than the other group.

While the studies described so far have pointed to direct effects of linguistic impairment on the communicative use of language, it is important to consider some possible indirect effects. Children may adopt strategies to compensate for their language disabilities. For example, they may fail to ask questions or to request clarification in order to avoid showing a lack of comprehension. Similarly, they may adopt defensive strategies in conversation, such as adopting a noninitiating role, possibly as a consequence of a history of unsuccessful communication (Rosinski-McClendon and Newhoff, 1987). This strategy would lead to a restricted range of pragmatic skills. So although there may be similarities between language-impaired children and their language-matched peers in their communicative use of language, the reasons for these similarities could be different, because compensatory strategies and an awareness of a lack of comprehension, rather than linguistic immaturity, could affect the pragmatic behavior of language-impaired children.

The use of particular linguistic and conversational strategies to compensate for language disabilities implies that children are aware of these disabilities. This view has been referred to as the "metapragmatic hypothesis", because it suggests an ability to stand outside of communication and assess or comment on one's communicative abilities and deficiencies (Donahue, 1987). Indeed, there is some experimental evidence that suggests that children who are language-learning disabled are remarkably sensitive evaluators of their own performance and of the behavior of their listeners (Donahue and Bryan, 1983).

2. The pragmatic skills of the language-impaired group are inferior to those of their language-matched peers

In the case of this outcome, language-impaired children are even worse in pragmatic skills than would be predicted by their language ability. For example, in the use of initiations and responses in mother–child interaction, language-impaired children have performed less well than their language-matched peers (Conti-Ramsden and Friel-Patti, 1984). Similar results have been reported in several other studies. Compared with younger children matched for language skills, language-impaired children have been found to produce a more limited range of communicative intentions (Shatz, Bernstein and Shulman, 1980 Fey, Leonard and Wilcox, 1981; King, 1989); they produced a significantly greater number of conversational dysfluencies, such as hesitations, self-repairs and abandoned utterances in a narration task (MacLachlan and Chapman, 1988); they produced significantly less simultaneous speech and more turn interruptions (Craig and Evans, 1989); and they produced more inappropriate and less sophisticated responses to requests for clarification in normal conversation (Brinton, Fujiki and Sonnenberg, 1988) or in a referential communication task (King, 1989).

These results would seem to imply that, for these children, pragmatic skills lag behind linguistic skills. There are two possible explanations. First, if we accept the hypothesis that pragmatic skills depend on the prior acquisition of linguistic skills, then it could be that these children, who have already acquired the linguistic skills, are simply delayed in the onset of the associated pragmatic skills. Of course, this explanation depends crucially on the hypothesis that linguistic skills precede and are prerequisites for pragmatic skills.

The second possibility is that these children are pragmatically impaired in a way that is distinct from and in addition to their linguistic impairment. Support for this view comes from studies that have shown that children are deficient in pragmatic skills in tasks where their syntactic and semantic ability should have been adequate. The tasks involved children's ability to adapt the form and content of their messages to the needs and feelings of their listeners. In these tasks, the children required the ability to recognize listener attributes and understand their significance for appropriately adjusted speech. This is a social–cognitive ability which is required in addition to the linguistic ability to produce the required forms. Pearl, Donahue and Bryan (1985) found that language-learning-disabled children had difficulty in a task that involved delivering bad news tactfully. So despite an adequate linguistic repertoire the children produced less tactful messages than their comparison groups, thus indicating a social deficit in the ability to predict and accommodate the feelings of others. Similar findings emerged in a study of polite requests and persuasive appeals, in which language-learning-disabled children made adjustments, thus demonstrating an adequate linguistic repertoire, but did not make the sorts of adjustments that were appropriate to their listeners (Donahue, 1981). Thus their problems seemed to be in understanding social relationships and appreciating the implications of different listener attributes for socially appropriate speech.

A qualitative difference in pragmatic ability would also seem to explain the results of a study of children's ability to request clarification of ambiguous messages when playing the role of listener (Donahue, Pearl and Bryan, 1980). Language-learning-disabled children were less likely than their comparison groups to initiate the repair of conversational breakdown, even though they had the ability, as indicated in a follow-up task, to identify inadequate messages. They had also demonstrated that they had the required linguistic skills to produce appropriate clarification requests. Donahue, Pearl and Bryan suggest that these children lacked an understanding of the conversational rule concerning the obligation of the listener to initiate repair of conversational breakdown. Furthermore, their previous history of communicative difficulties may have led them to assume that breakdown was due to their own inadequate comprehension skills.

This asymmetry between children's linguistic and pragmatic skills points to a specific type of pragmatic disability which is distinct from linguistic ability, so that the explanations for the children's difficulties would seem to lie elsewhere. For example, in a study of children with moderate learning difficulties, it was found that these children, compared with normally developing children matched for linguistic ability and mental age, produced inappropriate or no responses in a task involving the use of a range of speech acts, were unable to provide discriminating information or to request clarification of inadequate messages in a series of referential communication tasks, and were unable to impute beliefs to others and to realize that others' knowledge might be different from their own in a conceptual perspective-taking task (King, 1989). This type of pragmatic disability will be picked up in group design studies where the children are also language-impaired – their pragmatic performance will be equal to or inferior to that of their language-matched peers. What will not be picked up are those cases of children who are not language-impaired at all but who nevertheless have other deficiencies which give rise to a specific deficiency in the use of language for communication.

3. The pragmatic skills of the language-impaired group are superior to those of their language-matched peers

Here the suggestion is that children who are language-impaired may nevertheless have few or no problems with pragmatic aspects of language – in other words, that linguistic and pragmatic ability are not related. This would support the groupings of children into syntactic–phonologic and semantic–pragmatic groups. Children with syntactic–phonologic disorder would not be expected to have pragmatic problems. If this is the case, then examining the pragmatic skills of these children is unlikely to shed any light on the nature of pragmatic disability.

Some studies have in fact demonstrated that language-impaired children have pragmatic skills that are in advance of their linguistic skills, as indicated by their superior performance relative to younger language-matched peers in pragmatic tasks. Fey and Leonard (1983) report a study which found that in referential communication tasks the performance of language-impaired children exceeded that of their language-matched peers. Similar results were found by Meline (1986, 1988) in tasks involving the encoding of new information, while Donahue (1987) reports evidence that language-learning-disabled children demonstrated skilled pragmatic performance in terms of their recognition of the need to clarify their messages and in spite of syntactic deficiencies.

A possible explanation for these findings is that the language-impaired children, by virtue of being older than language-matched peers, have had more experience of situations requiring these communicative skills. For example, Donahue surmises that these children may have had greater experience of requests for clarification due to their language disorder. In other words, language disability in this case does not predict pragmatic disability – on the contrary, it gives more opportunities to develop pragmatic competence.

It is difficult to examine pragmatic ability without considering language, because language is involved in most communicative tasks. One study which addresses this separation investigated the conversational abilities of language-impaired children during the single-word utterance period of development, where it was possible to examine the children's conversational abilities without considering the role of syntax (Leonard, 1986). Children with language impairment (aged 2;10 to 3;6) were matched with younger normally developing children at the one-word utterance stage, ages 1;5 to 1;11, and their replies to an adult's questions, statements and directives in a conversational setting were analyzed. The language-impaired children used a greater range and greater sophistication of replies. Leonard suggests that two factors explain this finding. First, being older the language-impaired children were able to profit from their superior world knowledge and conversational experience in spite of their limited expressive skills. Secondly, as these children were more advanced than their language-matched peers in comprehension abilities, they were able to monitor more closely the utterances of their adult partners.

Studies such as these are important because they indicate that some aspects of pragmatic ability are unrelated to linguistic ability. This finding is similar to that discussed in the previous section, although with different consequences. In that case, children's performance in communicative tasks was inferior to that of language-matched peers, which suggests that they had a specific impairment in pragmatic abilities. In this case the children appear to have the social and cognitive skills required for the use of language in social contexts, despite their linguistic problems. These children, although language-impaired, should not be considered as having pragmatic difficulties.

4. The pragmatic skills of the language-impaired group are superior to those of their age-matched peers

There is little support for this position in the literature, and we would not expect it on logical grounds. However, it is possible that children who are otherwise impaired might excel in some aspect of communication that relates to their specific abilities or qualities, or to their conversational experiences. For example, Meline (1988) reports that his language-impaired group was more effective than age-mates as well as language-mates when using graphic descriptions to encode novel referents. Meline found that the graphic descriptions of the language-impaired group – for example, "It has four lines and they all have curves on them" – were longer and more detailed. A possible explanation is that these children were more patient describers of detail than the other groups of children.

Experience of conversational problems could also enable a language-impaired child to develop more sophisticated conversational skills than age-matched peers. One scenario might be as follows: a child who is language-impaired has to spend a lot of time repeating and clarifying his or her utterances in order to improve communication with others. This child would gain extensive practice in making clarifications. Thus, despite an inability to formulate the clarifications – which is predicted by the language impairment – the child might be aware of when clarifications are necessary and of how they contribute to mutual understanding. Such a child could then become superior to age-matched peers in this aspect of language use.

More generally, even though this fourth outcome is less plausible than the previous three, it should be noted that cases are frequently reported of children (particularly autistic children) who have pockets of ability far exceeding their performance in other areas. It would be worth looking out for such skills in children who are otherwise impaired because these skills may provide building blocks for remediation programs.

Summary: relating linguistic and pragmatic ability

From the studies discussed so far in this chapter, it is clear that there is often a relationship between a child's linguistic and pragmatic ability. This is only to be expected because the ability to use language must depend to some extent on a knowledge of language structure. There are, however, important aspects of pragmatic ability that are not related to knowledge of language structure and these are dealt with in detail in Chapter 6. Furthermore, even where there is some suggestion of a relationship between linguistic and pragmatic abilities, it must be clear to us what the nature of this relationship is. It is all too easy to assume that children first learn language structures and then how to use these structures. As shown later, this assumption has been questioned by functional linguists who argue that children's acquisition of linguistic structures is a consequence of their need to express themselves in communication.

More generally, there is the problem that work in this area is often impoverished theoretically. As Donahue (1987, p.162) writes:

> rather than randomly correlating aspects of syntactic–semantic knowledge with pragmatic development and then trying to come up with post hoc explanations, we must formulate a theory-driven model to derive hypotheses about the local effects of specific linguistic skills on specific pragmatic behaviors.

In relating linguistic to pragmatic ability, it is necessary to look closely at how the acquisition (or absence) of particular linguistic structures might affect a child's ability to perform particular communication acts. To do this, it is necessary to examine the correspondence between particular syntactic constructions and particular pragmatic skills. Some obvious examples are: the use of the definite article to mark information that is mutually known to speaker and listener; the use of interrogative constructions in certain types of request for action and in requests for clarification; or the use of relative clauses in providing more specific information about a referent. However, there are many cases where no clear correspondences are to be found. What, for example, is the syntactic correlate of a persuasive appeal or of the justification of a noncompliant response to a request?

Furthermore, in relating linguistic knowledge to the use of language, we need to be clear about what we mean by knowledge of linguistic constructions. In many studies a global estimate of syntactic ability is used

– in some cases, it is as global as MLU (mean length of utterance). Much more precise information is required, for example, whether the child uses a particular structure, such as relative clauses, for other functions but not for the function under investigation; whether knowledge of the construction is inferred from evidence of the child's linguistic production or comprehension; whether the construction is used spontaneously; or whether it can be traced to an imitation of some previous adult utterance (whether the imitation is partial, deferred, extended etc). In the absence of such information the claim that the child is syntactically competent is uninformative.

Finally, as already suggested, it is necessary to determine where the problem lies. If a child fails to produce polite requests, is it because of a deficiency in the required syntactic constructions, an inability to use them when required, or a lack of social judgment (for example, inability to assess listener attributes or to appreciate the implications of differences for socially appropriate speech)?

The complexity of these questions is seen when the findings of a study by Donahue (1981) are examined in which children were required to produce requests to listeners of different age or social status. Language-learning-disabled boys produced more polite requests to peers than to high-power targets as well as fewer and a smaller range of persuasive appeals. However, the fact that they made any adjustments at all demonstrated that they had an adequate linguistic repertoire. The fact that they produced different forms according to listener type also demonstrated that they had the social ability to perceive distinctive features of listeners. What they lacked was the ability to appreciate the implications of these differences for socially appropriate speech. In other words, the question of how to apply language knowledge in conversation requires an understanding of the social and sociocognitive issues involved – that is, a more complex theory than what is implied by a simple knowledge/use dichotomy. These issues are discussed in greater detail in Chapter 6.

Pragmatic factors and language learning

Up until now, the examination of the relationships between linguistic and pragmatic ability in children has involved investigating the ways in which linguistic ability determines the development of pragmatic ability. The other side of the coin is concerned with the ways in which pragmatic factors play a role in language development. It is important to consider the ways in which parental styles of interaction either help or hinder language learning in normally developing and language-impaired children. First a theory of language development is considered briefly – referred to as the *functionalist view* – in which the child's acquisition of particular linguistic forms is explained in terms of communicative functions.

The functionalist view of language acquisition

In the functionalist view of language acquisition, proposed by Bates and MacWhinney (1982), it is suggested that several grammatical structures – such as ellipsis, contrastive stress, and the use of pronouns and articles – are governed by the need for the listener to distinguish between old and new information in the discourse. Thus the development of grammatical structures is explained in terms of the communicative functions that the structures serve and, in particular, in terms of the child's active search for ways of expressing new functions using language. A further example would be the search for ways of making information in utterances more specific in order to take account of a listener's needs – such as using relative clauses and similar but more complex structures. However, despite the strong arguments that have been put forward for functional explanations of language development, there have been equally strong counter-arguments, particularly in the case of children's acquisition of those linguistic structures which are difficult to explain in functional terms – such as grammatical inflections and agreements (Karmiloff-Smith, 1979; Maratsos and Chalkley, 1981).

Parent–child interactions with normal language learners: what may help language learning?

Various lines of research on parent–child interactions have provided evidence to suggest that adults modify their communicative behaviors to accommodate the limited competencies of young language-learning children. With this support system, it appears that children can enter into conversation-like interactions with parents from very early in life and that from very early on they can achieve communication, sharing meaning and participating in joint routines. In Chapter 4 early prelinguistic development was discussed in detail. Early prelinguistic interactions provide a foundation for subsequent parent–child interaction involving language. A brief recap is given of those aspects of early prelinguistic interactions that contribute to this foundation.

Early prelinguistic interactions
Bruner's work (1978, 1983) has shown us ways in which parents and children evolve routines in the course of play and everyday caregiving. A routine is an established set of ordered, rule-governed, repetitive activities which provide the crucial support for the child to discover how to use language. Thus, a routine such as "peekabo" allows the infant to learn how

to take turns, how to perform certain actions and insert them in their appropriate slots in the conversational episode. In the same vein, Bates and her colleagues (Bates, Camaioni and Volterra, 1975; Bates, 1976) have shown that there are increasingly sophisticated uses of gestures by adults in parent–child interaction in the period just before the emergence of language. It is thought that the increased use of gestures facilitates the sharing of meaning by providing the child with an easier access to the symbolic communicative system. The work of Bateson (1975, 1979) and Trevarthen (1979), among others, has also pointed to the adjustments adults make in their behaviors to fit the abilities of infants in the first year of life. They have found that parents and infants can achieve patterns of finely tuned interaction where the temporal structure of their intercourse bears striking similarities to the format of conversations among competent language users – hence the use of the term "proto-conversations" to describe this phenomenon. Proto-conversations are possible because parents allow the infant to set the pace of the interaction and parents attribute intentionality to the infants' expressive contributions from the start.

Parentese

Another major line of research has been concerned with the verbal behaviors of parents towards their young language-learning children. The differences between child-directed speech and adult–adult speech are now so well known and well documented in the literature that the term "motherese", and more recently "parentese", has been coined to refer to them as a cluster of co-occurring behaviors. The emphasis on parents is purely coincidental in that most studies involved mothers, but it is now known that parentese is present in caregiver–child talk no matter who the caregiver is.

It is now clear that speech addressed to young children is higher in pitch, has a wider frequency range and has an exaggerated intonation pattern (Garnica, 1977); it is much simpler in both syntax and semantics as well as being more redundant, having fewer clauses per utterance, fewer modifiers per noun phrase, and more frequent repetitions and paraphrases of utterances (Snow, 1972); it is also slower, clearer and more fluent, having longer pauses between words and between utterances (Broen, 1972). In addition, parents frequently ask questions of their children, expand on what they say, and talk about the here-and-now (Snow and Ferguson, 1977). Thus, typical exchanges between mothers and their 20-month-old children are as follows:

Mother–son dyad
C: Car (looking out the window)
M: You see a car?
     (comes to window)
     A big car

C: Yeah
    Mine
M: Yours?

Mother–daughter dyad
C: That my ball
M: That is your ball
    Would you like to play?

Having described the characteristics of parentese, researchers began to question the role of these features in the acquisition of language.

Fine-tuning
A group of researchers proposed that parentese could be thought as being "finely tuned" to the child's own language level, that is, as the child's own linguistic ability develops, the caregivers decrease the amount of simplification and modification of their child-directed talk, thus always providing a sort of "scaffold" for the child to learn language. The early studies seemed to support this notion because differences were found in maternal speech to 2 year olds versus 10 year olds (Snow, 1972); between maternal speech addressed to 1, 2, and 3 year olds (Longhurst and Stepanich, 1975), and between maternal speech to 18 versus 28 month olds (Phillips, 1973). In these studies maternal speech increased in complexity as the children grew older.

Nonetheless, these early studies investigated maternal speech and child language development over large spans in development, thus only providing a measure of "gross-tuning". Consequently, a large number of correlational studies emerged to ascertain relationships between specific aspects of maternal speech and specific aspects of child language growth over shorter periods of development, but the results of these investigations were inconsistent and contradictory at times. In the area of maternal syntax and child expressive language, some investigators found no significant correlations between maternal MLU and child MLU (Newport, Gleitman and Gleitman, 1977; Gleitman, Newport and Gleitman, 1984; Nelson et al., 1984;) while others have found positive correlations (Cross, 1977) and, further still, negative correlations (Furrow, Nelson and Benedict, 1979). An examination of other relationships has also proven evasive. Of interest, however, are three findings. First, Nelson and his colleagues found some interesting correlations with specific aspects of maternal and child syntax. For example, they found that maternal auxiliary use to 27-month-old children was positively correlated with child auxiliary use at that time (27 months), and, that maternal auxiliary use to 22 month olds predicted child MLU at 27 months. These findings suggest that some aspects of adult speech to young language-learning children may be more sensitive than others and thus it is conceivable that we may find "fine-tuning" for certain aspects of care-givers' speech to children and not others. Secondly, Cross (1977) found that all of her significant correlations were stronger when she related maternal syntax and child receptive language ability, suggesting that mothers may be adjusting to their children's ability to understand more than to their ability to put words together. However, it has been found that the characteristics of speech to young children are also used by human beings when addressing their pets and plants (Hirsch-Pasek and Treiman, 1982), suggesting that other aspects of the child besides comprehension and production may well play a part on eliciting parentese. Thirdly, the work of Snow and her colleagues (Snow and Goldfield, 1983; Snow, Perlmann and Nathan, 1987) suggests that parents may adjust the syntactic complexity of their speech differently in different situations. Thus, routine situations such as book-reading have been shown to elicit more complex language than nonroutinized situations such as free play. These three important factors – that fine-tuning may be different for different aspects of parental speech, that fine-tuning may vary as to what aspects of the child the parent focuses on, and that fine-tuning may be situation-specific – all provide us with hints as to why there may be such a confusing pattern of results in the literature with normal-language learners. Presently as it stands, we can pick any position with respect to fine-tuning and find a handful of studies that will support our chosen position.

Semantic contingency

The problem of how the environment affects the young child learning language has also been approached from a different angle. It has been observed that parent–child interaction from early infancy through the preschool years is consistently child-centered; specifically, it has been found that caregivers respond contingently to children's utterances, often taking the child's own utterance and adding slight adjustments to make them more adult-like. Take the following examples from a mother and her 22-month-old daughter:

C: It yours (giving mother a cup)
M: It is mine

C: Want playdough
M: You want some playdough?
     Let's take the playdough out

C: Cup (handle comes off)
M: The cup broke

C: (brings a toy teddy)
M: A teddy bear!

The mother in the above examples responds by continuing with the central meaning in her daughter's previous utterances or behavioral acts (see last example). She often moderately departs in form from her child's previous utterance so as to provide an optimal chance for the child to see the discrepancy between her own linguistic system and the adult's. Since the original work of Cross (1978), this phenomenon of semantically contingent responses has been found to have a facilitative effect on child language acquisition. Thus, Snow (1982) found that vocabulary growth of children at the one-word stage was related to maternal use of semantically contingent responses to the children's focus of attention. Similarly, Wells and his colleagues (Barnes et al., 1983) found that semantically contingent responses strongly predicted language gain while Goldfield (1985) found that semantically contingent responses, as in the last example above where the mother names the object the child is showing, predicted the child's learning of nouns.

In contrast to the fine-tuning hypothesis, semantic contingency appears to be a robust phenomenon in child language acquisition research with English-speaking children. Experimental studies have also corroborated the original findings. Thus, Nelson and his colleagues (Nelson, 1977, 1981; Baker and Nelson, 1984; Nelson et al., 1984) have found that semantically contingent responses, especially recasts (a reply that structurally changes one or more components of the child's previous utterance but leaves the rest unchanged) facilitates the learning of grammatical structure, for example, the passive. Nonetheless, semantic contingency in parent–child interaction is not a universal phenomenon. Ethnographic studies by anthropologists have shown that other societies, such as Samoan (Ochs and Schieffelin, 1984), Kaluli (Schieffelin, 1984) and African (LeVine, 1977), do not have semantically contingent models for parent–child interaction. The children in these cultures nonetheless learn language. What does their environment provide for these children as a possible scaffold for language learning?

Routines
Snow and her colleagues (Snow, Perlmann and Nathan, 1987) have recently proposed that there may be two ways available to caregivers to build scaffolds for their young language-learning children. One is semantic contingency as described in the section above, the other involves building routines. In these routines, the caregiver imposes predictable sequences of actions accompanied by predictable language on the child often enough so that the child comes to recognize what the structure of these routines is. Some examples of these routines are games, nursery rhymes

and verses. The caregiver thus takes advantage of the predictability of the situation built by the routine to offer opportunities to learn language. This type of parent–child interaction is more adult-driven but has the same end result as semantic contingency, that is, of putting the child's utterance in context. Interestingly, it appears that parent–child interaction in routinized form is more frequent in other cultures other than American–European societies.

Before leaving this section on features of parent–child interaction that appear to function as possible positive catalysts for child language growth, it is necessary to clarify that none of the three aspects discussed above – fine-tuning, semantic contingency, and predictable routines – are mutually exclusive and they are not independent, that is, we should not conceive of these features as being options parents have to choose from and we cannot characterize the environment unidimensionally as "good" or "bad" with respect to one of the features. As Snow has clearly pointed out, these features may co-vary together, for example, speech that is highly semantically contingent need not be high on predictability, and speech that is highly predictable may not be contingent at a particular stage of development. Parents may choose to apply a contingency model for inter-action for one particular type of activity, or for a particular set of linguistic concerns, or at a particular point in their children's development. Similarly, they may decide to practice a different model of interaction based on predictability. Different cultures as well as special populations such as language-impaired children may restrict parents in their choices.

Parent–child interaction with normal language learners: what may hinder language growth?

It is a well-known fact that there is a great deal of individual variation in the rate of language acquisition in young children. Just as researchers have been interested in finding out how the environment may help the child to learn language, they have also been keen to find out what may hinder the young child's language growth. However, it must be clear from the outset that this research is concerned with individual differences in *normal* language-learning children and not with language delay as a clinical problem. Three lines of research have been concerned with this question and each is discussed in turn.

Rejection
Nelson (1973) argued that mothers' sensitivity was an important factor in young children's early language learning. She studied 18 mother–child dyads and focused on how the children learned their first 50 words. She found that her subjects fell into two categories: a referential group who

used mainly nominals (for example, *car*, *shoe*, *sock*) and an expressive group who used their first words mainly to express desires and refusals, and to control the behavior of others (for example, *more*, *no*, *bye*). Nelson then observed whether these children over-extended their first words, that is whether they used the same word to cover other meanings such as using the word *shoe* for *boot*. She then studied mothers' acceptance or rejection of their children's language: Did mothers follow the child's lead and accept the child's attempts to organize meaning and language or did mothers reject the child's novice attempts at producing the first 50 words? Those who were accepting were thought of as matching with their children's predispositions while those rejecting were thought of as mismatching.

Interestingly, Nelson found that the above dimensions contributed to the rate and smoothness of the young child's very early language development. Children who had shown a cognitive match with their mothers tended to begin to talk early and to continue to develop without much difficulty. However, children who had experienced a cognitive mismatch tended to start to talk later and sometimes had a period when they talked followed by a period of silence as if they were trying to sort out just how they were going to tackle the language-learning problem. Nelson made strong suggestions as to the possible long-term effects of rejection and suggested that a rejecting environment may well be a major factor in turning the child into a passive learner at a later stage. Nonetheless, there were major limitations with Nelson's study which caution us to moderate the interpretation of her results. First, only 18 children participated in the study and even with this small number many of the children had both expressive and referential characteristics in their early speech. Secondly, Nelson measured language growth in terms of vocabulary size and thus it is not surprising that those children who were referential had smoother rates of development because they were interested in objects to begin with. If social talk had been the measure, maybe the expressive children would have come out as having smoother developments than they did. Finally, although there is no doubt that sensitivity on the part of parents to their children's early linguistic attempts to engage in conversation is an important variable in the acquisition of language, our knowledge of discourse as a dyadic phenomenon throws the ball back into the child's court. It is not enough just to look at the parents and assess whether they are sensitive or not, it is necessary to look at the child and see what the child's contribution to the interaction is. The child's characteristics when engaging in dialogue may well create difficulties for even the most sensitive and well-motivated parents. This last consideration is of particular relevance when we try to evaluate the linguistic environment of language-impaired children.

Directiveness

A variety of studies with young normal language learners has suggested that parental speech used primarily to direct or control the child's behavior has been associated with a slower rate of language acquisition. Newport, Gleitman and Gleitman (1977) and Furrow, Nelson and Benedict (1979) both found in their longitudinal studies of 1 year olds that frequency of maternal imperatives ("Look here!", "Turn it this way!") was negatively correlated with children's gains in syntactic development. Cross (1978) and Demos (1982) also found this trend. Nonetheless the way in which directiveness is defined by the researchers is very important. Thus, Wells and his colleagues (Barnes et al., 1983) functionally defined directives as to the role they played in discourse, for example, the question: "Can you pass me the bear?" can, in the context of a mother talking to her child and extending her hand, function as an indirect directive for the child to give the bear to mummy and not to answer the question with a *yes* or *no*. With this definition they found a positive correlation between parental speech and children's language growth.

Other variables of interest are those that which appear to affect parental directive styles. Research indicated that low-socioeconomic status (SES) mother–child dyads engage more frequently in directive interactions (Bronson, 1974; Snow et al., 1976; Ramey, Sparling and Wasik, 1981) and that maternal education and IQ are negatively associated with the use of directives (Adams and Ramey, 1980). Once again, these variations were conceived as related to variations in the normal child's rate and smoothness of development and not to the presence of child language disorders.

Timing

The work of Harris and her colleagues (Harris, Jones and Grant, 1983, 1984; Harris et al., 1986), Roth (1987) and Stella-Prorok (1983) have all pointed to the importance of timing in parent–child interaction. For the young child learning language it appears that temporal delays in responding interfere with the young child's perception of contingent relationships. Thus, Harris found that in two groups of normal language learners, the slower developers participated in interactions where their mothers talked about an object before or after the child was attending to it. Thus, maternal speech was not related to the child's *current* focus of attention. Furthermore, Roth found that the lack of prompt maternal responses (within 1 second) to their 12-month-old children's vocalizations was related to decreased responsiveness on the part of the mother. Stella-Prorok experimentally introduced a 3-second delay interval to the conversations of an adult with 2 year olds and found that this temporal delay in responding completely disrupted the flow of the conversation and hindered communication. After a short time the 2 year olds stopped responding completely as if they could not handle this temporal delay despite the fact that the actual delayed responses were contingent, easy to process replies. Thus, it appears that children at the early stages of language learning suffer from the consequences of ill-timing of parental utterances.

The above three lines of thought point to different features of parental style which may negatively affect the smooth learning of language and, although conceived separately, many researchers have realized the close relationship between them. Thus, it has been noted that children of directive mothers appear to have a more expressive style of language. It was mentioned in the first section that expressive children appeared to have slower early vocabulary development. Similarly, it has been suggested that mothers who are directive do not temporally relate their replies to the infant's vocalizations or activities, that is, they are not closely related to what the child is doing or looking at. Maternal responses which function to control or direct the infant's behavior toward the mother's activities are not temporally contingent on the child's current focus of attention or activity; instead they interrupt that attention and activity and thus appear not to provide support for language learning. Conceivably then, these possible negative features can come together to form a "nonsupportive" environment for language learning. The success of all normal children in these studies in learning language points to the fact that young normal children can adapt to these environments and can develop language, albeit not always smoothly. The question then arises: Can language-impaired children do the same?

Parent–child interaction with language-impaired children

Research with impaired populations has typically lagged behind that of normal populations and language development has not been an exception. For clarity of presentation and discussion it would have been desirable to have had similar lines of research for language-impaired children to those outlined in the previous two sections for normal language learners, but this has not always been the case. In addition, other considerations such as the effect of the characteristics of the child on parental interaction have redirected the research questions almost midway. In what follows, there is an attempt to provide a comprehensive review of parent–child interaction with language-impaired children, pointing wherever possible to the similarities and gaps with respect to the above literature on normal language learners. For the purposes of this chapter, unless otherwise specified, language-impaired children will refer to those children who are having difficulties in the process of acquiring language but who are otherwise cognitively, emotionally, and physiologically intact.

Parentese

One of the most prevalent questions in parent–child interaction with language-impaired children has been whether these children receive input that is similar to that received by normal language learners, that is, do parents of language-impaired children receive parentese like parents of young normally developing children? The results of these investigations have been both limited and somewhat controversial, although if placed in historical perspective it is possible to trace an increasing awareness on the part of all researchers that the answer to this question may well be more complicated than originally conceived.

On the one hand, some researchers have argued that parental speech to language-impaired children is different from that of normal language-learning children (Buium, Rynders and Turnure, 1973; Marshall, Hegrenes and Goldstein, 1973; Wulbert et al., 1975; Bondurant, Romeo and Kretschmer, 1983) while, on the other hand, some researchers have suggested that maternal speech to language-impaired children is similar to that of normal language-learning children (Rondal, 1977; MacPherson and Weber-Olsen, 1980; Conti-Ramsden and Friel-Patti, 1983). What can account for such conflicting results? First, the clinical populations studied have not been comparable from study to study. The earlier studies tended to include in their populations of language-impaired subjects children with known cognitive difficulties and genetic abnormalities while the later studies attempted to control for the range of linguistic and cognitive difficulties of their subjects. Secondly, the control groups used to compare language-impaired children have been different across studies. The earlier studies tended to use chronological age matches while later studies matched for language stage using mean length of utterance (MLU) or they attempted to match for mental age. More recent studies acknowledge the fact that each of these comparisons is useful and can shed different light on the same problem. Thirdly, research with language-impaired children has seen a switch from more syntactic analyses of maternal input to more pragmatic analyses; thus it is not surprising that different results have been obtained.

At this stage in our understanding of parent–child interaction with language-impaired children it is clear that parents do use parentese when addressing their language-impaired children. The parentese they use is very similar to that used by parents of normal language learners of the same language stage although not identical because there may be variations in specific aspects of parentese which are significantly different from that received by normal language learners. These variations are usually related to the characteristics of the language-impaired child, for example, parents of severely language-impaired children may use simpler language when addressing their children (see Cross, 1984, for a review).

Interestingly, research has been limited to one particular design, that is comparisons between an experimental group of language-impaired children and a control group of normal language learners. Although the importance of such studies cannot be over-emphasized, we need to be aware that such studies only provide a partial view of the relationship between parental speech and child language problems. This research assumes that normal and language-impaired parent–child dyads function similarly and thus any differences found in some way predict or may exacerbate the children's language problem and should be decreased through intervention. This may indeed be the case, but it cannot be just assumed and it is necessary to demonstrate the exact relationship between specific aspects of parental speech and child speech in language-impaired children. A notable exception in this respect is the work of Lasky and Klopp (1982). These researchers began by reporting that mothers of language-impaired children used parentese in interaction much like normal language learners, but then they studied the associations between measures of the children's linguistic maturity and their mothers' parentese interaction patterns. Interestingly, they found that what appeared to be positively correlated with language growth for the normal language learners was not so for the language-impaired children. Thus, the same input may have different effects depending on the characteristics of the adult–child dyad. More intensive research with language-impaired parent–child dyads across time and in different contexts is very much needed.

Semantic contingency
Given the robustness of the findings that there are positive effects of semantic contingency on normal language-learning children's communicative development, it is natural that researchers interested in language-impaired children have asked a similar question of this population. Once again the research design has been one of comparison with the normal, and the results have not been unanimous in their conclusions. Some researchers have found that mothers of language-impaired children use fewer semantically contingent utterances than mothers of normal language learners (Newhoff, Silverman and Millet, 1980; Cross, 1981; Petersen and Sherrod, 1982; Horsborough, Cross and Ball, 1985) while other investigators have found that the linguistic environment of language-impaired children is similar, in terms of semantic contingency, to that of nonlanguage-impaired children (MacPherson and Weber-Olsen, 1980; Lasky and Klopp, 1982; Bondurant, Romeo and Kretschmer, 1983). Apart from the methodological considerations outlined in the section on parentese, there are other variables that may account for this discrepant picture. First, researchers are increasingly aware of the role of individual differences in their results. It is known that parents of language-impaired children vary as individuals with respect to their use of semantically

contingent speech. Thus, although group data may reveal certain differences or similarities, a closer look at the individual reveals heterogeneity: some parents behave very much like parents of normal language learners while others do not. Secondly, the issue of the comprehension status and age difference between the language-impaired children and the control group children is also currently being addressed. If researchers match for chronological age, there will be a language difference between the language-impaired children and the control group. If the researchers match for expressive language stage, then there will be an age gap and there may be a gap between the comprehension abilities of the two groups of children. If the researchers match for both expression and comprehension, then we have the presence of comprehension problems which may influence parental speech. There is no easy solution to the difficulty of comparing language-impaired and normal language dyads. We are acknowledging that comparability between dyads involving language-impaired children and normal language learners is not viable but then we have to continue with the research, controlling as many relevant variables as is possible and interpreting results cautiously. Another possibility that needs to be further exploited is research within the population of language-impaired children. It would be of interest, for example, to identify and compare different interactional styles in language-impaired dyads, deriving histories of interaction after following a variety of language-impaired dyads over time.

Finally, the effect that the child has on the parent has continued to be investigated by researchers interested in language-impaired children. In the area of semantic contingency, a recent study by Conti-Ramsden (1990) has shed some interesting light on this area. Conti-Ramsden studied 14 mother–child dyads with language-impaired children and 14 normal dyads. She concentrated on the use of recasts by mothers, that is, a reply that structurally changes one or more components of the child's previous utterance but repeats the rest. For example:

C: I mama's
M: You are at mama's?

C: Bill tractor
M: Bill has a tractor

These recasts have been thought to be semantically contingent replies par excellence in that they take the child's thought or focus of attention and they incorporate it into the parent's next utterance in the conversation, only this time it is an adult version. The presence of such sequentially contingent speech has been thought to trigger a procedure of comparison between the child version and the adult version and thus to help the child learn language (Nelson, 1977, 1981; Nelson et al., 1984). Conti-Ramsden then found that there was a significant positive correlation between maternal use of recasts and children's level of intelligibility. The more intelligible the language-impaired child was, the more her mother was able to use recasts. Thus, intelligibility in the language-impaired children helped their mothers to formulate recasts. This makes common sense because any person interacting with children needs to be able to understand what they intend to communicate in order to be able to take the linguistic form of their thoughts and put them in the adult version.

Thus fully intelligible and partially intelligible child utterances can hinder the ability of parents to be responsive and to reply contingently to their language-impaired children's communicative attempts. The following anecdote illustrates this point in its extreme. Laura, a language-unit teacher in the rural north of England, helps eight children with a variety of problems. Paul is a 6 year old with severe phonologic–syntactic difficulties. He is very fond of his teacher and has a routine of running to her in the mornings and telling her some item of news about what happened at home the night before. Laura admits that often she has a very hard time understanding what Paul wants to say. She may get part of his utterances, e.g. something about a car, but that is all. Thus, she usually tries to be responsive, but she often has to be rather vague and say "Oh, really?", "That's interesting", "I bet you enjoyed that". One day Paul came running and said something about his budgie and Laura said "I bet you enjoyed that" and smiled. Immediately Paul burst out crying. Laura felt awful. She later found out from his mother that Paul's budgie had died the night before.

The other side of the coin also needs to be pointed out. Parents of language-impaired children may have difficulties being semantically contingent due, at least in part, to their children's intelligibility problems. This explanation recognizes the influence of the children's difficulties on the parent. Nonetheless, the influence of the parent on the child is also present. No matter how hard parents of language-impaired children try to be responsive, sometimes they cannot be owing to their children's problems. Thus, parental language to language-impaired children may fail to reinforce their children's small steps towards acquiring the language system. In this sense, parental speech, and more generally any adult–child-directed speech to language-impaired children, may have the potential for exacerbating the children's problems.

Directiveness

One of the more consistent findings in the literature on parent–child interaction with language-impaired children has been parents' directive style. This has been measured in different ways by different researchers, be it increased use of imperatives (Buium, Rynders and Turnure, 1973), mands, that is, demands, commands and requests (Marshall, Hegrenes and Goldstein, 1973), or initiations in dialogue (Conti-Ramsden and Friel-Patti, 1983, 1984; Conti-Ramsden, 1990). A highly directive parent tends to use language primarily to control the child's attention and behavior, rather than using language as a reciprocal communicative exchange.

Possible reasons for these findings emerge from both partners involved in the dyad. From the parents' involvement, Newhoff and Browning (1983) have suggested that parents' knowledge that their child is disordered may affect their interaction in various ways. For example, the parents may no longer be able to gauge the linguistic level and needs of their children as the normal pattern of development has been disrupted and can no longer be used as a model. From the angle of the child's characteristics, Conti-Ramsden has pointed to two possible explanations for the increased directiveness of parents. First, the literature has consistently shown that language-impaired children are more passive in conversational interaction than their normal language-learning counterparts (Conti-Ramsden and Friel-Patti, 1983, 1984; Bryan, 1986), that is, they do not actively engage in conversational turn-taking and they do not initiate as often as normal language learners at the same language stage. Thus, it may be the case that in order to maintain a conversation with their language-impaired children, parents have to adjust their conversational style to be more directive and to initiate more. A second possible explanation comes from the attentional abilities of language-impaired children. Parents of language-impaired children may have consciously to direct their children's attention to their own as well as to their mothers' activities in order to achieve some level of involvement in the interaction. Fortunately, these possible explanations are all testable and researchers no doubt will be looking to investigate them more thoroughly.

Gaps in the literature

Various areas addressed in the normal literature have not been directly applied to the language-impaired population, for example, the work on early prelinguistic interactions of mothers and their young infants engaging in proto-conversations (Bruner, 1978, 1983). This is not surprising because language impairment is rarely identified at this stage of the child's development. Similarly, the work on timing of parental contingent speech (Harris et al., 1986; Roth, 1987) has mainly focused on young infants around 12 months of age, which once again has limited its applicability as a model for research with language-impaired children. To know how early parent–child interaction works with language-impaired children is desirable and it is particularly desirable for children with conversational disorders who appear otherwise normal. Because conversation appears to have its roots in early prelinguistic interaction, it is important that we try to assess in some way how this system worked for the conversationally disabled child. Unfortunately, at present our ability to identify children who present with conversational disorders in the presence of otherwise normal language is very limited. The earliest report has been of a 3 year old (Conti-Ramsden and Gunn, 1986), although more commonly research with these children has been understandably limited to school-age subjects (McTear, 1985a; Adams and Bishop, 1989; Bishop and Adams, 1989). A possible starting point could be to interview parents of conversationally disabled children in order to ascertain the flavor of their earlier interactions.

Another point of departure has been the fine-tuning hypothesis. This research with normal language-learning children has proven inconclusive and the correlational methodology marred with difficulties (see Gleitman, Newport and Gleitman, 1984, for a review). Thus, a strong parallel line of thought with respect to language-impaired children has not been in evidence. Similarly, the issue of rejection brought about by Katherine Nelson (1973) has not been followed in the same way as she conceived it, that is, for the very beginnings of expressive language (the first 50 words) and with respect to children's over-extensions. Instead, this idea has been translated into the use of disapproval, null-responses or rejecting utterances by mothers of language-impaired children. Some researchers have found that mothers of language-impaired children produce fewer acknowledgments and more generally negative responses but these have usually been related to these children's decreased ability to communicate effectively and have not always been replicated by other investigations (see Cross, 1984, for a review). Finally, routines have been investigated with respect more to models for intervention (Constable, 1983, 1986) than to natural parent–child interactions. No doubt this emphasis is being widened by current research.

Parent–child interaction revisited

The current state of our knowledge affords little guidance for the language-impaired parent–child dyad. It has been suggested that (1) normal language-learning children are exposed to a variety of interactive environments; (2) parent–child conversations with their normal language-learning children are quite different in character from culture to culture; and (3) different characteristics of parental language are likely to change depending on what aspects of the child the parent focuses on, what situation the parent–child dyad is engaged in, and at what language stage the child is. These facts taken together may bewilder us at first and push us to conclude that no language environment is better than any other for language learning.

Snow and her colleagues (Snow, Perlmann and Nathan, 1987) have suggested that the highly buffered nature of language learning, that is, its resistance to failure and the wide variety of successful language-learning environments available to the normal child, need not push us into the conclusion that the input language to the child is immaterial, but instead should lead us to recognize that it can work in different ways. The key and common ingredient in the variety of parent–child environments available to the normal language-learning child is the fact that adults create context around the child's speech. Children then actively extract from the input language information useful to the development of their own communicative system.

Research with language-impaired children has pointed to various complicating factors when we deal with impaired populations. First, language-impaired children may not be as skilled as normal language learners in their ability to extract, filter, organize, and use linguistic information and this in turn appears to affect parental input language. Secondly, features that have been thought of as possibly hindering language growth, such as rejection, directiveness and ill-timing, may all be circumvented by the normal language-learning child and result in normal language development, but the language-impaired child may not be able to do the same. In this sense, parental language style may be a factor in language-impaired children's rate of language development and this possibility needs to be investigated more thoroughly. Finally, it has been obvious throughout the discussion that features of parental language appear to be highly dependent on the language stage and other characteristics of the child. By definition, language-impaired children present a mismatch of characteristics to their parents in terms of their size, age, language ability etc., which may have stronger effects than have so far been contemplated.

The current state of our knowledge is also limited in that most of the work on interaction as described above, has concerned language–syntactic issues rather than pragmatic ones. The research on the verbal modifications of parents towards their young language-learning children has focused on finding a link between parental language and children's linguistic, and more specifically syntactic, advances, for example, it was argued that semantic contingency fosters syntactic growth while directiveness may not. Also, the different issues such as timing and fine-tuning are examined under a similar light. Nonetheless, recent interest in communication breakdown, repair and negotiations in parent–child interaction, which was reviewed in Chapter 4 in the discussion of clarification requests, has shown how interactional features may affect the child's developing pragmatic–communicative system and this area is gathering momentum in current research.

Concluding remarks

In this chapter relationships between children's linguistic abilities and their pragmatic development.have been examined, showing how some pragmatic skills are closely related to, or even depend on, linguistic ability. This information is important when considering assessment and intervention. If linguistic impairment predicts pragmatic disability, then it will be important to treat the child's linguistic problems first in the expectation that pragmatic ability will improve as a result. However, as seen in the examination of group design studies, which have investigated the pragmatic abilities of language-impaired children, the relationships between linguistic ability and pragmatic ability are not as clear cut as this. Indeed, it is possible for children to be language-impaired without any pragmatic disability, while it it also possible for children to be pragmatically impaired without any obvious linguistic deficiencies. This would suggest that there are some aspects of language use that are independent of linguistic ability, and that can be considered as specific pragmatic skills to be acquired in addition to the acquisition of linguistic structures. Turn-allocation and attention-getting are clear examples, while in other cases, such as speech acts and clarification requests, some aspects of the accomplishment of these functions depends on specific pragmatic knowledge. Furthermore, there are alternative explanations for pragmatic disability, such as cognitive impairment, sociocognitive deficiencies, and affective and emotional difficulties and are discussed in the next chapter.

This chapter has also examined the effects of pragmatic factors on children's linguistic development. The functional view of language acquisition was considered briefly – this suggests that children acquire linguistic structures because they have a need to express particular communicative functions. However, there are many aspects of linguistic structure that cannot be explained easily in this way. The literature on parent–child interaction was reviewed in detail, showing how some parental styles have been shown to be facilitative of linguistic development while others are detrimental. It will be important to bear these interactional features in mind when the questions of intervention are considered in Chapter 8.

Chapter 6
Alternative explanations

From what has been said so far, it has become clear that there is a need for a better understanding of what is meant by pragmatic disability. Indeed, what has emerged from this review of the research literature is that there are probably several different types of pragmatic disability, which may or may not co-occur in a particular child, and that the underlying causes of these different types may also be diverse. In other words, pragmatic disability would appear not to be a unitary phenomenon but to encompass a constellation of factors which adversely affect a child's use of language in communicative contexts.

As seen in Chapter 5, some of the problems that children have with the use of language seem to be primarily linguistic in origin, such as the inability to provide an accurate and discriminating description due to a lack of the necessary vocabulary and grammatical constructions. In these cases the child's difficulties with language give rise to problems in engaging effectively in communication. It was also seen how other problems may have little to do with actual linguistic ability but more with specific aspects of communicative competence, such as the ability to take turns in conversation, perform speech acts appropriately, or apply conversational principles such as the maxim of relevance.

In this chapter the following factors are considered which have been found to be related to pragmatic disability: (1) cognitive impairment; sociocognitive deficits; (2) affective and emotional difficulties.

Under cognitive impairment the more obvious cases of mental handicap and learning disability are examined first as explanations for pragmatic disability. However, there are less obvious ways in which cognitive impairment can affect the ability to use language in everyday conversation. Conversation is usually about persons, objects and events in the real world. The term "world knowledge" is often used to refer to all the information that we tend to take for granted but that we draw on to make sense of communicated information. Some children appear to have cognitive deficits affecting their commonsense world knowledge, so that their ability to make sense of what happens around them or to make inferences about implicit information is affected.

Sociocognitive aspects of communication involve the ability to take into account the needs and characteristics of the addressee so as to be able to construct appropriate messages. Some children appear to have deficiencies in sociocognitive aspects of communication, so that they are impaired in their ability to infer the beliefs and intentions of other people. This type of deficiency has been associated particularly with autism and the characteristics of autism relating to pragmatic disability will be considered in some detail.

Finally, there is also an affective aspect to communication, which is concerned with how communication relates to a child's emotional needs. Children's pragmatic difficulties may be explained in terms of affective problems, for example, previous communicative failures that can result in socially inept behavior, such as social withdrawal or inappropriate overfriendliness.

Cognitive impairment

Mental handicap

In recent years, the communicative abilities of mentally handicapped children have received considerable attention. A wide range of conversational skills has been studied including the use of communicative functions (Greenwald and Leonard, 1979; Owen and MacDonald, 1982), request–response rules (Kamhi and Johnston, 1982; Leifer and Lewis, 1984), conversational participation (Beveridge, Spencer and Mittler, 1979; Jones, 1980), and perspective-taking (Bliss, 1985), among others. In most ways the development of mentally handicapped children's communicative abilities has been found to run broadly parallel to those of non-handicapped children, albeit more slowly and with greater variability in speed of development, and with some notable differences such as playing a nondominant role in conversation (Kamhi and Masterson, 1989). As appears to be the norm in research, there is no clear answer as to whether mentally handicapped children are delayed or different; it appears that they may be both, depending on which aspect we are looking at and under which circumstances we study the phenomena.

Investigations with infants with mental handicap have noted that these infants are more passive in interaction. Mentally handicapped children do not initiate anywhere near as much as normal children do. Fischer (1983, 1987) found that Down's syndrome children initiated with vocal signals approximately 24 percent of the time compared with 52 percent for normal children of the same language stage. Similarly, Stoneman, Brody

and Abbott (1983) found that Down's syndrome syndrome children
tended to be less spontaneous, using significantly fewer child-initiated
verbal exchanges. Jones (1980) also found that Down's syndrome children
used referential gaze (child appears to be making some reference to his or
her activity by glancing up) less frequently. In addition, Eheart (1982)
found that mentally handicapped children responded less frequently in
conversational interaction and Leifer and Lewis (1984) further qualified
that these replies were much more often unrelated responses.

In recent years, the aforementioned observations have been interpreted
within the dynamic framework of interaction suggested in Chapter 3,
where influences are thought to be bidirectional: from adult to child and
from child to adult. Thus, studies of parent–child interaction with young
mentally handicapped children have suggested that parents of these
children tend to be less responsive and give less feedback (Jones, 1977;
Cunningham et al., 1981); and they more frequently assume a teacher-like
role in the interaction with frequent initiations and directives (Marshall,
Hegrenes and Goldstein, 1973; Terdal, Jackson and Garner, 1975; Petersen
and Sherrod, 1982). Nonetheless, recent research has pointed out the need
to look at individual differences and the role of early intervention in the
development of communicative competence in Down's syndrome
children. Fischer (1987), for example, found that although children with
Down's syndrome were less spontaneous in initiating social communication, their mothers were no more directive than mothers of
nonhandicapped children. Furthermore, mothers of the children with
Down's syndrome appeared to respond to more of their children's
communicative signals, especially if they involved vocalizations. Fischer
argues that early intervention programs may have fostered the mothers'
responsive, nondirective behaviors. In broad and general terms, however,
it seems that parent–child interaction with young mentally handicapped
children may be asymmetric and not always synchronous. This lack of
smoothness in the relationship between parents and their mentally
handicapped children is the result of the mutual characteristics of the child
and parent (Cardoso-Martins and Mervis, 1985). In a sense it is like a
vicious circle. The mentally handicapped child's lack of response results in
the parent trying to initiate more, thus adopting a more dominant role,
which in turn makes the child more passive. In effect, these interactions
lack equilibrium and there is a strong tendency to an imbalance in the
degree of control that the child and parent have over the way the discourse
proceeds.

As mentally handicapped children grow older they continue to play a
nondominant role in conversations (for reviews see Beveridge, 1989;
Kamhi and Masterson, 1989). Kamhi investigated how mentally
handicapped children interacted with normal children of the same mental

age and with an adult experimenter. Kamhi found that the handicapped and nonhandicapped children showed comparable abilities in various communicative measures analyzed including the use of requests and responses, topic maintenance, and communicative sensitivity to the different conversational partners. However, the mentally handicapped children talked less with the adult experimenter and they played a more passive role with the young normal children in terms of the number of requests they used. Owen and MacDonald (1982) also found little difference between Down's syndrome and nondelayed children in their use of different illocutionary acts. However, these researchers remind us that this is not always the case. Results of other investigations have suggested that mentally handicapped institutionalized persons have socially inappropriate and disordered communication with their peers and caregivers (Bredosian and Prutting, 1978; Prior et al., 1979). Abbeduto and Rosenberg (1980) also looked at different aspects of communicative competence in mentally handicapped individuals in naturalistic settings. They found turn-taking, expressing and responding to illocutionary acts, requesting clarifications, requesting more information, and maintaining and changing the topic to be developing well in mentally handicapped persons. Handicapped persons took turns at speaking; they quickly terminated instances where overlap occurred; they responded appropriately to their conversational partner's utterances; they spoke to give and receive information; they sought request for clarification of ambiguous utterances; and they cooperated in the establishment and maintenance of a conversational focus or topic. These naturalistic studies suggest that mentally handicapped persons are able to consider their listeners' needs and participate in basic conversational interaction without much difficulty.

Nevertheless, Kamhi and Johnston (1982) found fewer questions used by mentally handicapped children and Borys (1979) found that when they did use questions they tended to be more redundant ones. Bliss (1985), in the same vein, found that mentally handicapped children's perspective-taking abilities (what Kamhi termed "communicative sensitivity") increased in sophistication with increased mental age, from 6 to 12 years much like nonhandicapped children of the same mental age, with the exception that at the mental age of 6 years, the handicapped children performed better than the nonhandicapped group. Bliss suggested that the increased chronological age and social experience of the handicapped group was at least partly responsible for the results. This social experience or understanding of the different ground rules that apply in different situations has been termed "social cognition"(Light, 1979).

Beveridge (1989) argues that the social–cognitive approach captures the point that many thought processes have an inherently social origin. This is of particular importance in mental handicap because it allows us as clinician-researchers to place social and communicative experiences at the center of the study of these children's development. By implication, it is then possible to attempt to overcome intellectual impairment through communicative exchanges and it is also possible to identify intellectually handicapping processes that can exist across these children's development. Thus, Beveridge and Evans (1978) and Beveridge, Spencer and Mittler (1979) demonstrated a connection between mentally handicapped children's problem-solving abilities and their personality type. They found that inhibitable, as opposed to excitable, children tended to avoid potentially problematic situations and thus were reluctant to engage in social activities that provided essential learning experiences for them. For example, a teacher gives everyone in the class a task to do except for one child, but that child will not ask the teacher why he or she was not given something to do. Maybe it is not surprising that the children did not ask for help from their teachers. Beveridge and Hurrell (1980) found that more than 50 percent of the initiations made by mentally handicapped children to their teachers were not responded to, and this social experience in itself can be at the root of some of these children's difficulties. It is thus clear that the ecology of mentally handicapped persons will interact with their general intellectual ability to produce a different profile of language use from that of their non-handicapped counterparts.

Another interesting area of research with mentally handicapped individuals has examined their *referential communication* abilities. In Chapter 3 referential communication was discussed with respect to normal children's developing pragmatic abilities and it was pointed out how data from experimental studies complemented the view of the child's developing communicative system. Contrary to the findings of naturalistic studies of spontaneous conversations, research with mentally handicapped young people has suggested that non face-to-face referential communication tasks are particularly problematic (Longhurst, 1974; Beveridge and Tatham, 1976; Rueda and Chan, 1980). Researchers have found that the performance of mentally handicapped people in referential tasks is poorer than would be predicted on the basis of their mental age. In addition, it appears that mentally handicapped individuals are often unsuccessful in referential communication despite adequate linguistic ability to produce and understand the verbal descriptions needed for the task. In other words, their performance is poorer than indicated by their language stage. In this vein, Abbeduto and Rosenberg (1987) have suggested that mentally handicapped individuals' difficulties may stem not from a deficient communicative competence, but from failure to understand the requirements of the task.

Learning disabilities

The issues discussed above are also relevant for children with learning disabilities and, thus, will not be repeated here. Learning-disabled children have been described as young persons who show deficits in one or more of the processes basic to normal learning (Wiig and Semel, 1984). They comprise a heterogeneous group and may have a variety of problems accompanying their learning difficulties such as motor difficulties (for example, clumsiness), perceptual problems (for example, analyzing what they are seeing), and memory deficits (for example, retrieving information), among others. For the purposes of discussion it is interesting to note that learning-disabled children appear to experience problems in using language in social interactions with both handicapped and nonhandicapped peers and adults.

Guralnick and Paul-Brown (1986) studied the communicative inter-actions of 4- to 6-year-old learning-disabled children (referring to them as mildly retarded) in interaction with moderately and severely handicapped peers as well as nonhandicapped children attending a mainstream program. The results indicated that learning-disabled children were sensitive to the linguistic and cognitive characteristics of their conversational partners. Learning-disabled children, for example, used fewer information requests with the more handicapped partners than they did with nonhandicapped children. However, in a previous study, Guralnick and Paul-Brown (1984) demonstrated that the social status of learning-disabled children as perceived by nonhandicapped children was problematic. Normal children perceived learning-disabled and more handicapped children as being of a lower status and thus did not interact with them as equals. For example, normal children rarely asked questions of handicapped children. These findings suggest that perceived social status may be a considerable factor in the quality of communicative interactions that learning-disabled children experience with both handicapped and nonhandicapped partners.

The work of Donahue and her colleagues has been discussed at some length in earlier chapters and will only be highlighted here. Donahue and her colleagues have provided us with further evidence that the conversational problems of learning-disabled children stem from social–communicative difficulties. Donahue (1981) investigated the requesting strategies of learning-disabled children attending second, fourth, and sixth grades. She found that although learning-disabled children had an adequate linguistic repertoire of syntactic–semantic forms for representing requests of differing degrees of politeness, they were unable to appreciate the implications of listener characteristics for socially appropriate speech. Thus, learning-disabled children produced more polite requests to low-power listeners than to high-power listeners. In the same vein, Donahue, Pearl and Bryan (1980) examined language-disabled children's understanding of conversational rules for initiating the repair of a communicative breakdown. They demonstrated that learning-disabled children were less active in conversation requesting less clarification of inadequate messages than their normal counterparts. These researchers argued that learning-disabled children lacked social understanding of the conversational rules that govern communicative breakdowns and as a result of this they did not indicate to their conversational partners when a message had not been adequately specified. Also, Bryan et al. (1981) found learning-disabled children to be less able to initiate and sustain interaction when placed in a dominant social position of acting the role of a TV host interviewing a nondisabled child. Learning-disabled children asked fewer questions and were less likely to produce open-ended questions in the interview.

Similarly, Bryan (1986) has reviewed a series of studies which suggest that learning-disabled children have difficulties developing positive peer relationships. She found learning-disabled children to be nonassertive and deferential when compared to nondisabled children. In peer classroom interaction, for example, normal children tended to command and the learning-disabled children tended to comply. Learning-disabled children were thus less likely to disagree with classmates and less likely to argue for their choices (Bryan, Donahue and Pearl, 1981). Interestingly, this pattern changed when learning-disabled children were observed in outdoor, recreational activities. Bryan (1974) and Bryan and Wheeler (1972) found that learning-disabled children were more aggressive and hostile towards their peers, using more unprovoked negative statements such as "Better not kick me on the face".

The above results underline the importance of context. The differences and deficits exhibited by learning-disabled children may be due at least in part to the different social–cognitive–linguistic demands of various situations they are engaged in. It appears that the nature of learning-disabled children's problems is best understood as a difficulty in understanding the social demands of differing conversational situations which hinders them from being able to use linguistic knowledge in a pragmatically competent way.

Cognitive aspects of language use

It has been argued that the ability to use language depends on appropriate world knowledge. Indeed, as Ochs (1979, p.10) has written:

> An essential part of becoming communicatively competent is acquiring background knowledge that interlocutors (in one's speech community) take for granted.

Background (or world) knowledge is what enables people to make sense of what is said in a conversation by relating it to previous experience and by making predictions based on knowledge about objects and persons in the everyday world. For example, to be able to make sense of a story about everyday events, such as a shopping expedition, it is necessary to have some knowledge of what sequences of events are likely to occur, what the likely participants in the events will be, and so on. In other words, we need to have knowledge of what Schank and Abelson (1977) have described as *scripts, goals and plans*, or what Nelson (1986) has described as *general event representations*.

Event knowledge enables us to make sense of stories and events in everyday life in several ways:

- We can make predictions from what we have just heard to what we are likely to hear next and so constrain the range of possible next utterances, thus reducing the load on our processing capacity.
- We can make inferences from what we have actually heard to what is likely to lie behind what was said. For example, if we hear that someone went shopping, we can assume, without being told, that they are likely to have spent some money and acquired some goods in return.
- We can make sense of deviations from the normal course of events – for example, if someone has gone shopping and has returned empty-handed, we can assume that they were unable to obtain what they were looking for.
- We can re-organize our cognitive structures in the light of new experiences to provide more general or more detailed structures.

The relevance of recent work in artificial intelligence on world knowledge for an understanding of pragmatic disability was discussed in Chapter 2. There is also a wide range of evidence from cognitive psychology to support the view that world knowledge is used to assist language understanding (see, for example, Bransford and McCarrell, 1974). There is also more recent evidence that young children have well-organized knowledge about familiar events involving temporally and causally related sequences. Olson and Nickerson (1979) showed how children use world knowledge to aid their comprehension of stories. Another example would be the types of routine described earlier in which children learn how to greet, take leave, give thanks, as well as engage in other socially appropriate and culturally specific forms of behavior (Gleason and Weintraub, 1976). As far as conversation is concerned, Nelson and Gruendel (1979) have suggested that children have scripts for activities that they talk about and that these scripts enable them to conduct a more coherent dialogue. Where scripts are held in common with other children or adults, interaction is likely to be more predictable because some degree of mutual understanding can be assumed. Indeed, as Nelson and Gruendel found, there is considerable commonality among children in terms of their knowledge of familiar events involving causally related sequences. This knowledge is to be found in children as young as 3 years and, even though older children produced more elaborate scripts, these were based on the same basic scripts as those of younger children.

Children's narratives provide a good source of information about their knowledge of scripts. Eisenberg (1985) found that children as young as 3 years appeared to be dependent on script-like information when discussing past experiences in conversation. Furthermore, there was a developmental progression from an initial restriction to the general properties of an event to a later ability to focus on unique aspects. For example, in the earlier stage the child might describe a birthday party solely in terms of general properties of the event, such as presents, the birthday cake, blowing out candles. A few months later, more specific aspects of the event, such as what a particular child was wearing or the presents that the birthday child received, could be described.

In a study involving older children, Pace and Feagans (1984) uncovered some interesting developments in children's ability to use scripts to support their understanding of narratives involving familiar events. Children aged 5 years demonstrated superior comprehension of stories involving familiar events such as supermarket shopping, for which they were likely to have scriptal knowledge, than for less familiar events such as planting a garden. They were also able to compile lists of the most common events in a script and to go beyond the information provided in a story by supplying implicit information that had been omitted. However, younger children of preschool age and up to second grade were less likely to detect information that violated their expectations – for example, a story in which a mother bought a color TV in a supermarket instead of a bag of cookies. In this case the children seemed to tune in automatically to a script once the script was recognized and to disregard text-specific information that might conflict with their own knowledge and expectations. This finding indicates that children make use of script-like knowledge when interpreting narratives. It also shows that, as in other communicative tasks, younger children can be misled by their expectations and by their failure to attend to specific information in the text or context.

Cognitive deficits affecting the use of language

It has frequently been observed that some children have difficulty in processing extended discourse such as stories and in keeping track of topics during the course of a conversation, in spite of normal comprehension abilities when tested for words and isolated sentences.

One study that examines the effect of deficient world knowledge on a child's use of language is McTear (1989), which expands on the earlier case study (McTear, 1985b) to show how the child appears unable to discern connections between everyday events and to go beyond the surface characteristics of an action or an utterance to its deeper, underlying significance. The analysis was based on a conversation that arose during a description task involving a problem situation depicted on a card and based on an everyday social scene. In this case the picture showed a child standing on the doorstep of a house, looking rather lost and having emptied the contents of his pockets on the ground beside him. To understand the situation it is necessary to go beyond these surface details and make the inference that the child has lost his key and is unable to enter the house. However, the subject in the case study failed totally to make this inference and persisted in describing superficial details in the picture, such as the boy's pencil which was lying on the ground. It was only after considerable prompting that he was able to show evidence of understanding the picture.

What was interesting in this study was that, although the subject failed to make the required inferences to demonstrate an understanding of the situation, his responses were generally reasonable and appropriate on their own terms. For example, he inferred that the boy had lost his dinner money, was locked out and had to wait for his mother, and could try to get in by the back door. He was able to reason about everyday events and to understand relationships between events at a local level – such as losing the dinner money and not being able to have dinner – but was unable to integrate these isolated pieces of knowledge into a larger coherent structure.

In order to appreciate this point, it is necessary to examine what knowledge is required to understand the event depicted in this task. In the present case, the fact that the child is standing outside the house leads to the inference that he has the goal of entering the house. However, this is not a logical inference and it could be cancelled on the basis of subsequent information. For example, the child may have been looking at the house because he heard a noise from inside, while emptying the contents of his pockets on the ground may have been due to something unrelated, such as looking for his bus fare. However, in the absence of this information it is usual to make the default inference that the child has the goal of entering the house. This being so, and given that he seems unable to achieve his goal, we can assume that there is some problem – for example, there is no one at home or he has lost his key. We can see each of the actions in this scene as having various preconditions and effects. For example, to be able to enter a house a person either needs a key or there should be someone to open the door. To use a key you have to be able to find it. To find it you may have to look in your pockets – and so on. McTear (1989) presents a goal tree setting out some of the knowledge about entering a house on which a child would have to draw to understand the depicted situation. As only some of the information is represented in the picture, it is necessary to use world knowledge to infer that information which is implicit. The subject in this case study appeared to be deficient in this ability to reason about implicit information.

Of course, a lot of questions are raised when we begin to consider the relationship between a child's world knowledge and language use. How has the child come to have deficient world knowledge in the first place?

To have world knowledge means that we have symbolic representations of states and relationships in the world. It is generally agreed that these representations are experientially derived. Nelson (1986) surmises that initial representations are first derived through immediate perception, but that they are constrained by our prior knowledge. These initial representations are then the content of subsequent cognitive operations – such as pattern analysis, categorization, inference and transformation. This analysis yields more abstract cognitive structures which will subsequently be used as a basis for the analysis of novel experiences. This process is illustrated in Figure 6.1.

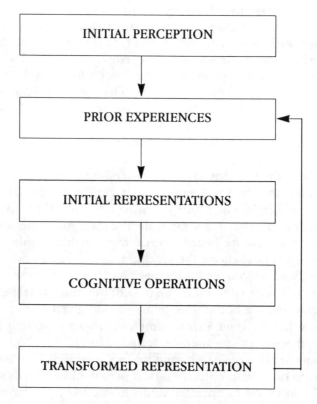

Figure 6.1 The acquisition of event knowledge

As we can see, there are a number of places where things can go wrong. There may be problems with the initial perception of an event. However, as this initial perception is constrained by prior knowledge, we have to go further back to examine this prior knowledge and how it was acquired. In other words, we are forced to ask whether the problem is one of limited world experience (which would affect an infant's understanding of a novel event) or whether it is a processing problem, such as an inability to perform the required cognitive operations of categorization, inference etc. This in turn raises the question of whether these abilities are innate or acquired. Further problems concern the ability to reorganize old knowledge structures in the light of new experience (what Piaget calls assimilation and accommodation), as well as the ability to retrieve the correct structures when required.

As might be imagined, an understanding of these issues requires a comprehensive theory of understanding. Most work in cognitive psychology focuses on components of such a theory without reference to the whole theory. Very little work has been carried out in speech pathology in relation to these issues, so this is an area where fruitful cooperation is possible between speech pathology, cognitive psychology, and artificial intelligence.

Sociocognitive deficits

Sociocognitive aspects of language use

In order to participate effectively in conversation a person has to be able to make social inferences about the actions, beliefs, and intentions of other persons in order to understand the behavior of others and to be able to adapt messages to their needs.

There is a growing interest in the relationships between social cognition and language use (Durkin, 1987). One aspect of developmental work in social cognition is concerned with how children conceptualize and reason about their social world (Shantz, 1983). The ability to make social inferences, that is, explanations of the underlying causes of another person's behavior, is essential for a full understanding of communicative processes. Two main traditions of research are relevant to this question: studies of children's role-taking abilities, and recent research on the development in children of the "theory of mind".

There are different levels of social inference. The most basic level involves the ability to recognize social attributes of listeners and to adjust messages accordingly. The studies of Donahue and colleagues suggest that children who are language-learning-disabled are able to vary requests according to differences in listener status, although boys seemed insensitive to differences in age when giving instructions to peers and younger listeners (Bryan, 1986; Donahue, 1987). However, more research is needed on this aspect of communicative competence.

As discussed in Chapter 3, there is a large literature on children's role-taking abilities, involving experimentally based studies of referential communication. These studies have typically demonstrated that young children are less able than older children to take the listener's knowledge into account in their communication – for example, when describing a picture – and that when required to make judgments following observations of communication failure, they tend to attribute blame to the listener rather than to the speaker's inadequate message. Studies have indicated that language-learning-disabled children are less likely to convey information that is appropriate and adequate. These problems may be due to linguistic impairments or to an inability to assess the listener's requirements and provide a description that is informative.

Theory of mind

The most sophisticated level of social inferencing has been investigated in studies of the development in young children of a "theory of mind", which enables children to infer mental states such as beliefs and intentions from the observable behavior of other people and to make predictions or adjust their messages on the basis of these inferences. While research on social cognition and role-taking is concerned with children's knowledge of all kinds of internal states, including emotional and motivational as well as cognitive states, recent work on "theory of mind" is concerned only with cognitive and volitional states – that is, with the ability to recognize mental states such as beliefs, knowledge, intentions, and desires, both in self and in others. The term "theory of mind" is used because these mental states are not directly observable. However, a theory of mind is essential for effective participation in social interaction because the ability to make inferences about the mental states of others enables a child to understand and make predictions about the behavior of other people.

There are a large number of studies concerned with how a theory of mind develops in young children (see, for example, papers in Astington, Olson and Harris, 1988). Furthermore, recent work on pragmatic disability, and in particular attempts to explain the pragmatic deficits of autistic children, has focused on what happens when a child appears to have a poorly developed or deficient theory of mind.

The basic principle underlying children's acquisition of a theory of mind is that around 2 years children begin to distinguish between the world (the way things are) and their mental representations of the world. Mental representations involve relationships between people and the world – for example, believing that it is raining, wanting the rain to stop, intending to work in the garden. The earliest evidence that children are beginning to acquire a theory of mind comes from two sources – their pretend play and their use of mental constructs. Around the age of 2, children begin to be able to engage in pretend play. For example, they might pretend that a banana is a telephone. In order to do this, they have to disconnect (or decouple) their representation of the banana as a telephone from their representation of the banana as a real object in the world. Thus two representations are involved – the secondary representation of the banana as telephone and the primary representation of the banana as real object, and the child is able to distinguish between these representations when engaging in pretend play (Leslie, 1987). Furthermore, at about the same time, children begin to use mental terms such as *know*, *think*, *remember*, and *forget*.

The most important development, as far as social interaction and communication is concerned, is the ability to use mental constructs to make explicit reference to what others believe, want and intend in order to predict and explain their actions and beliefs. This ability enables children to realize that other people often have beliefs, wishes and intentions that differ from their own. In turn, this knowledge enables children to distinguish between appearance and reality and between intentions and actions – distinctions that are essential for successful participation in social action.

One of the earliest developmental studies examined the ability of young children to infer mental states from observable events and to use these inferred states to make predictions about behavior (Wimmer and Perner, 1983). In particular, in this study the children were required to distinguish between what they themselves believed to be true and the false beliefs of another person. The experiment, which is often referred to as the *Sally–Anne story*, involves two dolls: Sally and Anne. Sally has a basket and Anne has a box. Sally has a marble and she puts it in her basket. She then goes out. Anne takes out Sally's marble and puts it into her box while Sally is away. When Sally comes back and wants to find her marble the critical question is asked: Where will Sally look for her marble? The correct answer is "in the basket". This is because Sally put it there and she has not seen it being moved by Anne. Sally thus *believes* that the marble is where she left it.

To succeed in this task, the subject has to distinguish between his or her own beliefs and the false beliefs of the other person. In this case, the child knows that the marble is in Anne's box, having seen Anne put it there. However, the child also needs to know that, as Sally has not seen Anne move the marble, Sally will continue to believe that it is still in the basket. Wimmer and Perner found that most 4–5 year olds responded incorrectly by predicting that Sally would go to the actual location of the marble (Anne's box), while most 6–9 year olds correctly predicted Sally's false belief (i.e. that the marble was still in the basket).

It will be helpful at this point to introduce some terminology. The term "first-order representation" has been used to describe representations that people have of objects and categories in the world (Leslie, 1987). "Second-order representations" involve mental representations about first-order representations – for example, thinking and reasoning about the content of our own and other people's minds. Second-order representations, which are the subject of the Sally–Anne experiment, involve the ability to represent a mental state – for example, to believe that another person has a belief or intention. Thus in this experiment the child is required to represent his or her own beliefs as well as the beliefs of Sally. The ability to do this enables the child to understand the behavior of others and to predict their behavior in particular situations, as in the experiment. The ability to form second (or higher)-order representations is sometimes also referred to as *metarepresentational ability*.

Higher-order representations are important for understanding social interaction because they involve the concern that people have about each other's mental states – for example, what a child believes the other person believes about the child's beliefs or intentions. An example will help to illustrate higher-order states (Perner and Wimmer, 1985).

Children were told stories in which two characters (John and Mary) were independently told that an object had been unexpectedly transferred to a new location. For example, an ice-cream van, which both knew was originally in front of the post office, had been moved to the town hall. Both John and Mary would know that the van was now at the town hall, but would not know that the other person knew this. So John's higher-order belief about Mary's belief would be incorrect – that is, John believes that Mary believes that the van is at the post office (and similarly for Mary's belief about John's belief). Perner and Wimmer found that it was not until the ages of 7–8 years that children could reliably make the correct judgments involving such higher-order mental states.

The ability to represent mental states is important for social interaction – for example, when distinguishing between a speaker's intentions and what they say. Second-order states are necessary to judge when a person is mistaken – that is, they have a false belief. However, higher-order representations are required to distinguish between a lie and a joke. In the case of a lie the speaker wants the listener to believe that what the speaker says is true, while the speaker believes it to be false. In other words, a deceptive speaker wants the listener to think a false statement is true. In the case of a joke, however, the speaker does not expect the listener to be misled, because both know that the statement is false and both know that the other knows this is the case.

In summary, children begin to acquire the ability to distinguish between the world and their representations of the world at about 2 years. They become able to infer the mental states of other persons from observable events or from communication, and to distinguish between their own mental states and those of others. More complex social understanding, such as distinguishing between a lie and a joke or understanding the role of beliefs and intentions when making judgments of moral responsibility and social commitment, develops later (around the age of 8). Similarly, more complex uses of language, such as irony and sarcasm, develop late because they depend on attribution of higher-order beliefs and intentions (see Perner, 1988, for further examples).

One potential puzzle is how children are able to engage effectively in communication if they do not acquire the necessary higher-order beliefs and intentions until they are 5 or 6 years old. In Chapter 4 it was seen that children as young as 9 months engage in intentional communication, in as much as they engage in behavior with which they intend to have an effect on a listener and persist in that behavior until the effect is achieved or failure is clearly indicated (Bates, 1979, p.338). However, it is necessary to distinguish between the child using behavioral clues about the effect on the listener and the attribution of a mental state to the listener. Young children can operate successfully with behavioral clues by making the assumption that beliefs and intentions are transparent. Thus they can engage effectively in normal, cooperative communication without having to engage in sophisticated analysis of intentions and beliefs. It is only when they become involved in more complex interaction, involving mistaken beliefs, deceptions, false promises, jokes and sarcasm, that they require an understanding of higher-order intentions and beliefs (Perner, 1988).

Sociocognitive deficiencies

It is being increasingly recognized that autistic children are particularly deficient in the ability to infer the mental states of others (Baron-Cohen, Leslie and Frith, 1985; Frith, 1989a). This deficiency has wide-ranging implications for communication, because communication depends on speakers and listeners being able to take account of each other's mental states. Indeed, it appears that due to this deficiency autistic children, while being able to produce syntactically correct utterances and even to vary their language as a function of gross social attributes of their listeners, fail to use language meaningfully and communicatively (Baron-Cohen, 1988). Thus autistic children are likely to violate the maxims of conversation postulated by Grice. Being unable to infer accurately their listener's knowledge, they will have difficulty with the maxim of quantity, which requires that we say no more and no less than is required. Similarly with the maxim of relevance, which requires that we make our utterances relevant to the needs of the listener. However, before looking at recent studies of autism in terms of the *theory of mind* hypothesis, it will be useful first to examine more generally the communicative difficulties faced by autistic children.

Autism

If any group of disordered children has as its central characteristic their inappropriate use of language for communicative purposes, it is autistic children. Since Kanner's (1943) description of autism, there has been a great deal of research in this area; Humphreys (1987) suggests that during the period 1984–1986 alone approximately 531 articles on autism were published. There are now substantial amounts of information on this area available but, due to space considerations, it is possible only to highlight the more salient features specifically related to pragmatics and social interaction.

Experienced clinician-researchers interested in autism have suggested that careful questioning of parents reveals subtle differences in the social–communicative development of autistic children from very early in life (Aarons and Gittens, 1987). For example, autistic infants may be described as "very good babies" because they are not demanding. They tend to fail to initiate and respond to social contact and do not reach out to be picked up. They may lie undisturbed for long periods and do not appear to be interested in parents or familiar people. Similarly, researchers have noted that autistic infants do not take part in the reciprocal "proto-conversations" discussed in Chapter 4 (Olson, 1970; Howlin, 1980) nor do they engage in the range of babbling and sound play normal infants do (Ricks, 1975). As development continues, these children experience difficulties with the interpretation of facial expressions, gesture and body language. Although some autistic children remain mute, many develop language, albeit usually very delayed. Once language develops, Tager-Flusberg (1981) points out that there does not appear to be a global language deficit in autism that affects the different aspects of linguistic functioning similarly. Instead, it appears that autistic children master phonology and syntax but exhibit major difficulties in semantic and pragmatic functioning.

Communication problems in autism

The characterization of conversational interaction with autistic children has received much attention, but there is yet to be a consensus with respect to the various types of pragmatic ability and disability involved in autistic children of different ages and severity. In general, it has been reported that autistic children use fewer initiations and that these initiations are often inappropriate. For example, Baltaxe (1977) reported that the adolescent autistic children in her study tended to ask the same question over and over again, despite having received an answer. Similarly, Hurtig, Ensrud and Tomblin (1982) found that questions by autistic children were used frequently and most of the time as devices to initiate interaction. These questions, however, were inappropriate or irrelevant to the topic being shared. Autistic children appeared to be using questions to obtain a response from the conversational partner and thus engage in interaction, but they seemed unable to select appropriate content for them. This last study suggests that some autistic children have some communicative intent as well as some ability to recognize the discourse expectations of certain conversational devices. A series of studies has also noted that autistic children's interactions fail to take into consideration the listener's perspective. This is a particular area of weakness for these children which has effects on conversational processes such as re-initiations, and the use of politeness forms and requests, among others. Thus, Ricks and Wing (1975) noted that autistics tend to speak too loudly in public places while Baltaxe and Simmons (1977) noted that these children seem to have major difficulties differentiating casual from polite forms of address for different conversational partners. Nonetheless, Fay and Schuler (1980) noted that some autistic children are able to rephrase initiations in order to get something they want. Autistic children may add "I" and "please" to their initiations or they increase the volume and pitch of their requests.

The construction of conversations necessitates a willing and responsive partner. In this respect, autistic children have also been noted as having major problems. Many autistic children are echolalic and echolalia can be thought of as a very low level of response. In echolalia the autistic child repeats the speaker's preceding utterance rather than providing a reply. Interestingly, Paccia and Curcio (1982) demonstrated that comprehension difficulties may be related to echolalia in communicative exchanges with autistic children. These investigators found that the more complex the preceding utterance, the more likely autistic children were to reply with echolalia. For example, wh-questions were more likely to be responded to with echolalia than utterances that required only to fill the gap, such as "The boy has an (apple)". The possible relationships between comprehension and conversational difficulties need to be further explored. Further findings indicate that autistic children have difficulties speaking on topic, that they tend to talk ad nauseum about topics that interest only themselves (for example, specific times in train schedules), and that they produce pseudo-dialogues where they themselves take the speaker and listener roles leaving no time for their conversational partner to ask questions or make responses.

Much like research with other populations, research with autistic individuals has benefited from experimental as well as from naturalistic studies. In the former category, the work of Hobson and colleagues needs to be noted. Hobson (1986a,b) and Hobson, Ouston and Lee (1988a,b) carried out experiments involving the recognition of emotional expressions in autistic and mentally handicapped individuals. The paradigm that they used involved the presentation of a stimulus, for example, a photograph, a schematic face, a voice, or an action sequence. These stimuli represented four emotional states: happy, sad, angry, and afraid. The task for the child involved matching a given presentation with one of the four stimuli. The matching was always across modalities. Thus, an angry looking picture had to be matched with an angry voice rather than a sad or afraid voice. The results of these studies suggested that autistic children are significantly impaired in their recognition of emotional states relative to their nonverbal mental age. In addition, autistic children have been found to have difficulties sharing attention (Landry and Loveland, 1988) and in the spontaneous use of expressive gestures such as hiding one's face in embarrassment (Attwood, Frith and Hermelin, 1988).

Although in this section some sort of a picture has been built about autistic individuals' communicative profiles, we have no way of distinguishing those features that appear at the core of the syndrome of autism and those peripheral features that may or may not be present in different individuals. At present there is immense individual variation in children diagnosed as autistic: Can we identify some key characteristics that may serve as the first step towards an explanation of the disorder?

Core problems in autism: Wing's triad

The problem of discovering the core problems of autistic individuals led Lorna Wing and her colleagues (Wing and Gould, 1979; Wing 1981a,b, 1988) to abandon the idea of a discrete syndrome of autism and instead advocate thinking in terms of a continuum or spectrum of autistic disorders. At the core of the *continuum of autistic disorders* lies an impairment of social interaction and it is this impairment that is the key to diagnosis. Wing further suggests that children with this social impairment are characterized by a triad of common and invariant features involving: impairment of social recognition, impairment of social communication, and impairment of social imagination. These characteristics are being referred to as "the triad of impairments of social interaction" or "*the triad*" for short. It is thought that these three impairments give rise to different kinds of behavior at different ages and at different stages of development. It is also recognized that in each of the three domains, a wide range of severity of impairment is present. Briefly, *impairment of social recognition* involves an inability to recognize other human beings as the most rewarding features of our environment, and ranges in degree from total aloofness and indifference to other people to subtle difficulties in getting to know people which are difficult to detect on brief acquaintance but are evident in longer contact. *Impairment of social communication* involves interacting with people through the medium of language. Impairment in this sphere ranges from complete absence of a desire to communicate with others to talkative children who engage in conversation but do not take full account of the reciprocal nature of interaction. For example, these children may ask inappropriate questions of their conversational partners. Finally, *impairment of social imagination* affects the ability to copy another person's actions with genuine understanding of their purpose and meaning. Thus, the development of symbolic and pretend play is affected especially when it involves putting oneself in the position of another person and experiencing thoughts and feelings. Once again the range of behaviors under this aspect of social impairment is wide. This aspect of the triad can vary from total lack of recognition of other people's feelings to the ability to recognize them in an intellectual way but without empathic sharing of emotions.

The range covered by the continuum of autistic disorders is enormously wide and covers pretty much all possibilities from profound mutism and isolation to normal eccentricity in social interaction. The most important causes of variation have been found to be chronological age and mental age (Wing and Attwood, 1987). Autism is rare in the normally intelligent population and very frequent in the mentally handicapped population. Independent evidence also exists which shows that normally intelligent autistic individuals may suffer from other neuropsychological disorders (Rumsey and Hamburger, 1988) and conversely that specific medical conditions can lead to autism (Coleman and Gilliberg, 1985). These findings lend support to Wing's (1988) thesis that a particular area of the brain is responsible for social interaction involving the three features of the triad and that problems in this area of the brain are what leads to its dysfunction. Consequently, the triad and its possible neurophysiological basis are seen as primary causes in the continuum of autistic disorders and not as secondary manifestations of other impairments such as language disorders. In addition, the presence or absence of the triad even in its mildest forms is seen as indicating social impairment and thus belonging to the continuum of autistic disorders. In this sense, the concept of a continuum or spectrum does not in any way imply a watered-down view of autism as a disturbance with recognizable characteristics but instead strengthens the basis from which "classic" autism and other difficulties stem. The assumption that there is a particular area of the brain responsible for the triad, but not for any other handicaps, forces us to look toward a single explanation for the disorder. Such a deficit would eventually be mapped onto the brain system that is affected. Recently, Wing's triad has been explained in terms of a single cognitive deficit – the absence of a theory of mind.

Explanations of autism: the theory of mind

Earlier there was discussion of how normal children develop a theory of mind and begin to recognize that they themselves and others think, pretend, believe, doubt, and imagine; that there is a distinction between the world and mental representations of the world; and that they can use this information to understand the intentions and feelings of others. The distinction was also made between first-order and second-order represen- tations, and the explanation given that second-order representations involve the ability to think and reason about one's own and other people's beliefs and intentions.

The hypothesis that autistic children lack the capacity for second-order representations and thus do not have an adequate theory of mind has been proposed as the single-fault explanation for the triad of social impairment (Baron-Cohen, Leslie and Frith, 1985). Frith (1989a,b) argues that this is a very powerful and specific hypothesis. It is powerful because it can explain through a single cognitive deficit the three aspects of social impairment that form the core of the continuum of autistic disorders. It is specific because it not only specifies where some if not all the problems must lie but also it specifies a whole important area that should remain intact, that is, first-order representations in perception, thought and language. A series of studies followed to gather evidence to support this hypothesis. In the original paper, Baron-Cohen, Leslie and Frith (1985) used the Sally–Anne story described earlier to study the development of a theory of mind in young children. Baron-Cohen and his colleagues used Down's syndrome and young normal children as controls. It is important for the theory of mind hypothesis of autism that the deficit only apply to autistic children and not to other groups such as the mentally handicapped – thus the need for control children from other handicaps.

Most of the nonautistic children gave the correct response but 80 percent of the autistic children gave the incorrect answer and said Sally would look in the box. Baron-Cohen, Leslie and Frith (1985) argue that these results support the hypothesis that autistic children fail to mentalize – that is, they cannot construct second-order representations and thus attribute mental states to others.

In 1986, the same researchers published a second paper based on the same three groups of subjects, this time using an original method to assess autistic children's ability to attribute false beliefs to others. The task involved asking the children to put four pictures in order to make up a story and to tell the story in their own words. Some of the sequences were mechanical, that is, one picture showed a child loosing a balloon, then the balloon flying away, then the balloon nearing a tree, and finally the balloon popping on a tree branch. Some of the sequences were behavioral, for example, a child walking down the street, getting to a sweet shop, paying some money and receiving sweets, and then leaving the sweet shop with sweets in hand. The third type of story, and the most crucial type, was mentalistic stories. These stories followed the logic of the Sally–Anne story and involved attribution of false beliefs. For example, one sequence showed a boy putting a chocolate in a box, going out to play, his mother comes in, finds the chocolate and eats it, the boy comes in and looks in the box for the chocolate (falsely believing that the chocolate would still be there) but does not find it. The results replicated their 1985 findings. Approximately 80 percent of autistic children were not able to sequence the story correctly and, in addition, used significantly fewer mental state terms in their narration than did the control groups.

In 1987 two important pieces of work furthered the hypothesis. Leslie (1987) made a distinction between pretend play and functional or reality play as the basis for his argument that pretence involves second-order representations and thus is at the basis of autistic children's lack of pretend play. Baron-Cohen (1987) set out to test this proposal and indeed found support for it. Furthermore, Baron-Cohen has continued to work to specify further the theory of mind hypothesis of autism. In his most recent research, Baron-Cohen suggests that autistic children's meta representational problems can not only explain autistic children's problems in attributing mental states to others but can also explain their difficulties with the appearance–reality distinction (Baron-Cohen, 1989a) and their insistence on repetitive behavior (Baron-Cohen, 1989b).

There is no doubt that the work of Baron-Cohen and colleagues has provided a great deal of insight into the possible reasons for the existence of the triad of social impairment in the autistic continuum. However, the theory of mind approach has not gone without its critics. Boucher (1989), for example, argues on methodological and logical grounds that a metarepresentational deficit is more likely to be a secondary rather than a primary all-explaining deficit in autism and instead proposes a primary motivational factor as responsible for the different characteristics of autistic people. Baron-Cohen (1989c) argues against the motivational explanation on the grounds that we still have to explain why autistic children are not motivated to use a theory of mind. Further research will no doubt continue to refine our thoughts in this area.

To conclude this section, it should also be noted that an inability to infer the mental states of others may occur with other groups of children beside autistic children. In their experiments, Baron-Cohen, Leslie and Frith (1985) compared autistic and Down's syndrome syndrome children and found that only the autistic children had difficulty with the task (the Wimmer and Perner (1983) experiment described earlier). However, King (1989) compared normally developing children, matched both for chronological and mental age, with children with moderate learning difficulty on this task and found that the latter group performed very poorly. More research is required involving carefully designed experimental tasks such as those used in these studies to assess the extent to which children who are described as having pragmatic disability are impaired in conceptual perspective-taking, and to assess the ways in which this impairment affects their communicative competence.

Affective and emotional difficulties

Affective aspects of language use

It was indicated in Chapter 4 how, in early interactions with caregivers, infants develop a motivation towards persons that is essential for dialogue. There has been a tendency to emphasize the cognitive and sociocognitive aspects of communication, looking at the content of communication and how it relates to the goals, intentions and beliefs of the communicating parties. However, there are affective aspects of communication that should also be considered. People often engage in dialogue, not primarily to exchange information, but to share experiences, solicit support, or to develop and sustain relationships with other people. On the one hand, communication provides emotional rewards, while at the same time the motivation to engage in communication with others depends on positive experience of such rewards. Furthermore, given that communication is reciprocal, there is a need for social sensitivity or empathy – the ability to take account of the emotions and feelings of others – which parallels the sociocognitive aspects described earlier, involving the ability to take account of the mental states of others. There is some evidence of a relationship between children's communication disorders and their emotional and behavioral problems, which is examined below. First, however, a brief outline is given of some aspects of the affective development of normally developing children, indicating how these aspects have a bearing on language use.

Affective development

In Chapter 5 it was discussed how researchers view parent–child communicative interaction as the basis from which language learning stems (Snow and Ferguson, 1977). Nonetheless, relatively little work has concentrated on individual family styles and specifically little attention has been paid to differences between families which might explain differences in the speech of children. This is particularly the case for the role that parental speech may have in determining the child's emotional or affective development (Bretherton and Beeghly-Smith, 1982). Interestingly, researchers interested in psychological theories of child development have yet to bridge such theories to parent–child language. There is a dearth of data relating to the ways parents use language to convey to their children concepts relating to emotions.

There is little doubt that the ability to interpret and understand the emotions of others is important not only for personality development, but especially for the development of *social competence*. To be socially competent and sensitive involves the ability to perceive and interpret correctly the moods and feelings of other people based on manifestations such as facial expression, tone of voice, and body posture. There appears to be a great deal of variation in this *social sensitivity* to others (Hoffman, 1981).

Social sensitivity is part of an individual's empathic ability and empathy in turn lies at the basis of responsiveness. It is thus surprising to find out how little we know about how these emotions are acquired. What researchers have concentrated on is what children appear to know about the emotions and feelings of others, that is, their *social cognitions*, rather than how they acquire this knowledge. Typically, studies have taken pictures depicting a variety of scenarios such as a boy losing something and have asked children of different ages how the child in the picture feels. Results suggest that children appear to label happiness and sadness more easily than fear or anger. Why this is the case is not clear.

Further work on the development of emotion has revealed that early in life, in the first 6 months, infants display many reactions that are suggestive of affective states, but it is unlikely that they involve conscious emotional states. For example, infants will widen their eyes, open their mouth and may have an increase in heart rate at the sight of a new, attractive object. Kagan (1984) argues that such states should be kept within the context in which they occur and derive their meaning from such context. Thus, an infant may be experiencing "surprise to novelty" and not emotions such as "happiness" or "delight". In the second part of the first year, new emotional reactions appear as a result of the maturation of cognitive functions, especially retrieval memory (Kagan, 1984). Emotions such as "fear of the unfamiliar", "protest "and "resistance" appear at this stage.

During the second year children continue to develop their emotional states, but at this stage it is also of interest to note that children begin to attempt to share plans and meanings with others (Garvey, 1977). Between the ages of 3 and 4 years, children develop the ability to assume that in interaction their listeners share their basic knowledge about events and the world around and shortly after these young children begin to use language to label basic emotions such as "sadness" and "happiness" (Bretherton and Beeghly-Smith, 1982). Interestingly, at this stage children also develop the ability to respond empathically to others (Zahn-Waxler, Radke-Yarrow and King, 1979). Later, during the sixth and seventh years of life, children begin to evaluate their own characteristics with those of others, leading to feelings such as "confidence", "insecurity", "pride" or "inferiority". At this stage the role of siblings and peers is very important because it provides the background against which the comparison of the self is made giving rise to changes in mood and behavior (Kagan, 1984).

Much like the nature versus nurture argument familiar to those interested in language development and disabilities, the study of affective development has also two major themes as its base. On the one hand, researchers argue that an innate biological package determines both the recognition and expression of emotions. On the other hand, others put socialization and interaction with the environment at the center of children's learning to identify and empathize with the emotions of others. There is no doubt that the controversy will continue. What is clear, however, is that, as a child develops, knowledge plays a more salient role in the expression and understanding of emotions. During the first years of life emotions are generated most often by external events, but by 7 years of age thoughts have become critical and emotions are dependent on ideas. As a result, emotional states are easier to change in younger than in older children and the adult is characterized by fewer changes in emotional states, more stable moods and feeling states, because these are not dependent on external stimuli produced by changes in the environment, but mainly on belief systems developed over childhood and adolescence.

Affective and emotional difficulties

Investigators interested in the relationship between communication and affect and in how affective and emotional difficulties affect children's ability to interact and communicate socially, have tackled the problem by looking at special populations (for a review see Prizant et al., 1990). On the one hand, they have looked at children with emotional–behavioral problems and ascertained the incidence of communication problems within this population (Baltaxe and Simmons, 1988). On the other hand, researchers have taken a population of language-impaired individuals and investigated the incidence of emotional–behavioral difficulties these children might have (Baker and Cantwell, 1982; Cantwell and Baker, 1985). Both approaches have found an association between communication disorders, emotional disorders and behavioral disorders, in children and adolescents.

Baltaxe and Simmons (1988) found a high incidence of language problems in child psychiatric populations. The figures vary in the literature but it appears that around 75 percent of children who present to psychiatric institutions also have communication or learning problems (Cantwell and Baker, 1985). Similarly, Cantwell and Baker also found that of 600 children with speech and language difficulties, 50 percent had a diagnosable affective or behavioral problem. This figure rose to 86 percent when children with learning as well as communication difficulties were included in the sample. Interestingly, both approaches have also noted qualitative differences. Baltaxe (1977), for example, noted that autistic German-speaking children had problems with the more pragmatic aspects of language use than with speech intelligibility or grammar. Thus, she found that autistic children confused the polite and familiar forms of address in German (*Sie* and *Du*), a confusion that may arise from a lack of understanding of social roles. She also documented turn-taking difficulties and problems with taking the listener's point of view in terms of marking new and old information in conversation.

In the same vein, Baker and Cantwell (1982) found that certain types of communication difficulties were associated more often with emotional–behavioral disorders than with others. In their sample, those children who were having communication problems as well as diagnosable emotional–behavioral problems were children who presented with language difficulties as opposed to speech difficulties. Their analysis of these distinctions was rather crude but, nonetheless, they were able to conclude that language use, comprehension, and processing appeared to be the more prevalent problems for children with communication and affective disorders. Conversely, however, Camarata, Hughes and Ruhl (1988) found that their group of children with behavioral difficulties had mainly language difficulties which could be described as syntactic rather than semantic in nature. Unfortunately, the authors used a tool that looked mainly at syntax which may have thus biased their results. The authors themselves conclude that a pragmatic analysis would have been desirable. There is no doubt that further qualitative research is needed in this area.

From the above findings four major hypotheses have arisen:

1. Emotional–behavioral disorders cause communication difficulties.
2. Communication difficulties cause emotional–behavioral disorders.
3. Both communication difficulties and emotional–behavioral disorders are related to each other because they are both related to some factor that causes both of them.
4. Communication difficulties and emotional–behavioral disorders are interrelated because they are both aspects of the developing individual. The child is in continuous interaction with the environment and the environment in turn affects the child. For example, a child may develop a difficult temperament which affects mother–child interaction. This may result in a reduction of mother–child interaction which in turn may lead to language delay.

Interestingly, there appears to be evidence that supports each of these possibilities. How can this be the case? The key lies on the type of emotional–behavioral disorder we are looking at, the heterogeneity of special populations, and the type of communication difficulties we are concentrating on. Most researchers today would agree that a relationship exists but it is early days in terms of defining the nature of this relationship. Further investigations are needed in this important area especially in the light of the current interest in pragmatic disability.

Concluding remarks

In this chapter some alternative explanations of pragmatic disability have been explored which do not rely on a close relationship between a child's acquisition of language structures and the ability to use language in communication. These alternative explanations involved looking at children's cognitive, sociocognitive and affective development and impairments, and explaining their pragmatic disabilities in terms of these factors. The relationships between pragmatic disability and specific disorders were also examined – in particular, mental handicap, learning disability, and autism.

The review of explanations of pragmatic disability in this and the preceding chapter leads to the confirmation that pragmatic disability is not a unitary phenomenon. As suggested earlier, there are different types of pragmatic disability. This would seem to make sense, because pragmatic ability – or the use of language in communication – involves a variety of skills. It has been shown how *linguistic impairment* can affect a child's use of language. However, there are other aspects of language use – referred to as *specific pragmatic skills* – that have little to do with linguistic ability and more to do with specific principles of communication. *Cognitive skills* – or the ability to represent world knowledge – determine the extent to which children can make sense of what is said to them and can communicate coherent information. *Sociocognitive skills*, which involve the ability to represent the mental states of others, are necessary for the construction of messages appropriate to the needs of listeners and for predicting the behavior of other persons in different situations. Finally, *affective and emotional factors* determine the nature of a child's relationships to other people and attitudes to communicative encounters, and have a bearing on the extent to which the child's communicative behavior is socially acceptable.

As shown, impairments in one or more of these aspects of communication will result in the sorts of behaviors that have been grouped together under the label *pragmatic disability*. However, it is important to emphasize that it is essential when assessing pragmatic disability and devising appropriate treatment programs to consider the possible factors involved, because a failure to look for explanations will result in a superficial approach that is less likely to be successful. The question of intervention in the light of these remarks is returned to in Chapter 8. First a look is taken at ways of assessing pragmatic disability.

Chapter 7
Assessing Pragmatic Disability

Pragmatic considerations in assessment

When confronted with the task of assessing an individual child's communicative system, be it at the phonologic, syntactic, semantic, or pragmatic level and involving either comprehension or production, it is necessary to take into consideration our current knowledge of what has been called broad pragmatics (see Chapter 1) and our understanding of an interactive framework for viewing the developing child (see Chapter 3). A narrow view of pragmatics is seen as an additional level of language above phonology, syntax and semantics – a level that needs to be assessed in its own right. This aspect of assessment will be discussed in the next section. A broad view of pragmatics, however, necessarily permeates the assessment of all language-impaired children because it is concerned with:

– the integration of linguistic structure and pragmatic rules;
– the study of situational effects on the use of language;
– methodological issues of data collection, transcription and analysis.

Similarly, the interactive framework discussed in Chapter 3 emphasizes the inter-relationship between the child and the environment underlining the importance of the dyad as the minimal unit of analysis.

Three major implications can be drawn from a pragmatic approach to the assessment of communication disorders in children. First, the realization that language is fundamentally an integration of structural and pragmatic knowledge and that communication also involves the integration of linguistic, social, and cognitive knowledge (Prutting, 1982; Prutting and Kirchner, 1983) has brought home to all of us the importance of natural language use. Children use language mainly when they feel the need to communicate and it is in this context that they need to be assessed. Clinicians have long been aware of the generalizability problems brought about by decontextualized intervention where structures are taught without regard to their content and use (Leonard, 1981). This same idea is now being applied to assessment. It is necessary that we collect valid, representative and relevant data about the child's communicative strengths and weaknesses and the pragmatic perspective suggests that this cannot be done successfully without paying attention to the child's ecology. Naturalistic assessment is now the most central element of the whole assessment procedure. Clinicians may well want to use standardized tools, interviews, tasks etc., but the information gathered in this way, which usually comprises a categorization of what the child can and cannot do, needs to be integrated within a pragmatic framework that emphasizes an interactive approach in order to understand how the child's communicative behaviors are related to one another (Muma, 1983). Thus, we need to develop and refine the tools available to clinicians to enable them to gather, systematically describe, and understand natural communicative interaction. Indeed, speech–language pathologists have always believed in the value of "an informal chat" with the child and parents. This informal chat, which usually took place at the beginning or end of the session, is now assuming the central core of our assessment protocols.

Second, assessment cannot involve one member of the dyad only, be it the child or the adult (usually a parent). Communication is an inter-actional, interpersonal process and as such it involves as a minimum two people: the dyad. Thus, we can no longer view communication disorders in children from an intrapersonal perspective, trying to find out what is wrong with the child's communication so that we can help that child overcome it alone. We need to consider the important roles significant others play in facilitating or constraining communication because the effects are always bidirectional, from child to significant other and from significant other to the child. In Chapter 3 a framework was provided for the development of the possible interactive alignments experienced by the child. This framework provides us with guidelines as to appropriate contexts in which assessment should take place. Thus, for example, assessment of a very young child should include caregiver–child interaction and the assessment of a young adolescent should include adult–child and child–child peer contexts.

Third, assessment of any particular aspect of language needs to amalgamate the contribution of pragmatic knowledge with the contribution of structural–semantic knowledge. Thus, at an initial assessment visit, a failure on the part of the child to produce a particular syntactic structure, in the clinic, with the clinician as the conversational partner, signifies that the child is not able to produce that particular syntactic structure, in a strange environment (the clinic) and with a nonfamiliar conversational partner (clinician). It does not necessarily mean that the child does not have that structure in his or her linguistic system, nor that, given a different context, e.g. with a parent at home, this structure will not be used. The opposite situation can also occur. In a home visit, a clinician may note comprehension on the part of the child to parental use of commands involving "before" such as "Before you go to bed, brush your teeth", or "Before you sit for dinner, wash your hands". This observation tells us that in parent–child interaction at home and with reference to everyday, repetitive, routine activities, the child understands structures referring to the order of events in time. This does not necessarily mean that the child's linguistic system is such that it can cope with this type of information nor that, given different structural–semantic information, e.g. the sentence "Before you touch the red block, touch the blue block", the child will be able to understand. Assessment thus has to be more comprehensive in that it always needs to integrate the pragmatic factors in the situation with the structural–linguistic knowledge necessary to participate in it.

Assessing pragmatics

A narrow view of pragmatics has brought forward an additional set of skills that are the concern of speech–language pathologists. Clinicians are actively seeking information about how children acquire the rules necessary in order to use language appropriately in a variety of contexts and how these skills are learned and used by language-impaired and other atypical populations. This additional set of language skills which the child acquires during development also needs to be assessed and understood within the interactional framework discussed in the previous section. Narrow pragmatics needs to be understood within broad pragmatics.

Prutting and Kirchner (1987) suggest that the paradigm necessary for conceptualizing pragmatic aspects of language is only just evolving and currently much of what is available involves the beginning stages of fact-gathering and description. This, nonetheless, should not hinder us as clinician-researchers from actively trying to apply what we know in order to assess pragmatics in language-disordered populations. As will be seen in this Chapter, procedures, materials, and tests are being developed to help the clinician provide a profile of the pragmatic abilities and deficits of different groups of language-learning children.

A distinction can be made between three main approaches to the assessment of pragmatics: the ethnographic method, the checklist approach, and the standardized test. Each of these approaches is examined in the following sections.

The ethnographic method

Ethnography refers to a method of study of events and persons in which one of the main aims is to discern underlying rules and patterns that operate for the participants (Ripich and Spinelli, 1985). The ethnographic method can be seen as an alternative to more traditional approaches to assessment in which the main focus is on the results of assessment – for example, the number of times a child performs a task correctly. In the ethnographic approach, however, the emphasis is on the processes of assessment – for example, how the child seems to arrive at a particular task performance, especially in cases where the child's answers are incorrect.

The ethnographic approach can be characterized in the following ways. First, it is *inductive*. What this means is that the analyst makes observations of a subject in selected contexts, collects data – for example, in the form of transcripts of interactions – and draws conclusions from a careful examination of the data. Thus the method requires keen observation skills and the ability to generalize from particular examples. A second characteristic is that the method involves *qualitative* as opposed to quantitative analysis. Rather than being concerned with the number of times a subject performs a particular action, the analysis involves a detailed examination of how the action gets performed. Thirdly, the approach is *naturalistic*, which means that it is considered important to observe events in their natural settings. Thus, if a child is reported as having difficulty with communication in everyday settings, it would not be considered sufficient to observe the child's behavior while interacting with a speech–language pathologist in a clinic; instead, it would be necessary to observe the child in a variety of contexts which reflected the child's everyday communicative situations. A fourth aspect is that the analyst needs to be able to *adopt the perspective of the subject under analysis*. In the case of a child with pragmatic disability, this would involve a child-centered perspective in which an attempt would be made to view the communicative context from the viewpoint of the child. This perspective contrasts with the more normative view typical of an adult-centered approach in which the child's performance is measured against norms of expected or desired behavior. Thus, instead of judging a child inadequate due to the failure of the child to use a particular communicative skill in the way that a child of the same age or an adult would do, the analyst examines the way in which the child actually uses the skill in question and attempts to assess its effectiveness (or lack of effectiveness) in terms of the child's perspective. The identification of avoidance strategies in children who have linguistic and communicative difficulties owes much to this more child-centered approach to analysis. Finally, the ethnographic approach is *constructionist*. What this means is the analyst examines the processes of an event rather than its outcome. In the case of an interaction involving an adult and a child, the emphasis would be on how both adult and child actively contribute to the interaction that evolves, rather than treating the interaction as directed by one of the participants – usually the adult.

Ripich and Spinelli (1985) outline an ethnographic approach to classroom assessment and intervention which could be generalized to the study of interactions in the clinic as well as of everyday situations outside the clinic in which the child is involved. Their approach consists of the following stages:

- identify the child to be studied, on the basis of reports, questionnaires, checklists, or referrals from people involved with the child, such as parents, teachers, or clinicians;
- make a preliminary description of the communicative problem based on these sources of information, which may be supplemented by interviews with the people concerned, including the child;
- develop a summary of the problem;
- observe the child in the relevant communicative contexts;
- summarize the observations and identify patterns of communication breakdown;
- validate these observations in consultation with the teacher, parent, or clinician and the child.

It might be useful to summarize a case study which Ripich and Spinelli (1985) present as illustration of the ethnographic method. The child they examined was unable to follow classroom instructions and had a low level of participation and attention in the classroom. The initial step of identification of the child and his problem was taken by the child's teacher. Next the clinician set about describing the communication problem, asking the teacher to elaborate on the nature of the problem as well as interviewing the child. The interview with the teacher was structured around a Classroom Communication Checklist (Ripich and Spinelli, 1985, p. 209), in which the teacher was asked to rate the child's effectiveness across a number of parameters, such as participation, manner and frequency of interruptions, ability to maintain attention and follow instructions, questioning, and descriptive ability. This information was supplemented by more specific information concerning different contexts in which the child's particular difficulties were observed. In this particular case, for example, it was found that the child never responded in whole class contexts, seldom participated in reading group discussions, and was more interactive in one-to-one situations.

In the interview with the child, each area of communicative breakdown was discussed and an attempt was made to elicit from the child the possible motivations for his behavior. The following example illustrates how some useful information was gained on the child's perspective to classroom participation (Ripich and Spinelli, 1985, p .209):

Clinician: Why do children not always answer in class?
Child: They don't know the answer or they don't think fast enough.
           My mum says it's better to listen.

Clinician: So do you try to listen?
Child: Yeah, that's the best way.

On the basis of these initial observations, the clinician concluded that the child's low level of classroom participation was due to the fact that he had over-generalized the rule that it is important to listen, while his difficulty with following classroom instructions was possibly related to processing difficulties. These conclusions were then tested and supported in classroom observations, following which it was concluded that the child only communicated when highly motivated – for example, when he needed information to complete his work, and that his difficulties in following instructions were due partly to the way the teacher presented the instructions as well as to his processing difficulties. These problems were intensified in larger groups. The observations were validated in further interviews with the teacher and the child and options for a plan of intervention were discussed, which involved the teacher attempting to be more systematic in giving instructions and the child practicing "doing his work right and talking more in class". Indeed, the intervention strategy that was implemented involved developing the child's ability to make clarification requests appropriately, thus facilitating both classroom participation and attention.

The ethnographic approach has been described in some detail because it illustrates the strengths as well as the weaknesses of this method of assessment. One general point is that it is difficult to assess communicative skills outside of natural communicative contexts. The ethnographic method provides a way of overcoming this problem. It is important to emphasize that what is involved is not just a set of good observation skills, but rather the ability to generalize from these observations and to avoid being biased by prior assumptions. In this way it is possible to focus on the particular problems of an individual child, without having to interpret these problems within a predetermined theoretical framework. However, the other side of the coin is that the approach lacks generality because it cannot benefit from knowing what typical problems children encounter. It is for this reason that several investigators have developed checklists of pragmatic skills which observers can try to identify as they watch the child interact.

Checklists of pragmatic skills

Checklists serve to heighten the clinician's awareness of pragmatic issues which arise in everyday conversational interaction. Typically a checklist requires the observer to note the number of times a set of behaviors occurs in an interaction or sometimes simply whether it occurs or not. This can be done while the interaction is taking place, but more usually audio or video recordings are used so that a more accurate and a more easily verifiable analysis can be made.

There are now several checklists available for the analysis of pragmatic behaviors. A selection of these checklists is examined, and their strengths and weaknesses are summarized (for a description of a wide range of pragmatic assessment procedures, see also Smith and Leinonen, 1991). Following this, an assessment is made of the usefulness of checklists in general as a method for assessing pragmatic ability and disability, and some problems with the use of checklists are outlined. First two procedures are considered that are used to elicit information from parents and others interacting with a child about the child's communicative behaviors – in other words, reports about the child's communication. Afterwards checklists are examined which are used to analyze recordings and samples of actual communicative situations involving children. Both types of checklist are potentially useful as sources of information about a child's communicative abilities.

Pre-assessment Questionnaire
The Pre-assessment Questionnaire (Gallagher, 1983) is an attempt to address the problem of obtaining a representative sample of a child's language, given that a child's language performance varies across different contexts. These contexts may include the child's communicative partner or physical context variables such as the activities or materials used to elicit language samples. The Questionnaire is used as a means of obtaining information about the child's use of language in these different contexts from parents and other significant persons in the child's life.

The first part of the procedure is concerned with basic information, such as children and adults who live in the child's home. The next part includes questions about the nature of the child's communicative difficulties, based on reports of different persons. There follow questions concerning how the child's behavior changes when interacting with different partners – friend, younger and older sibling, teacher, mother, father, familiar adult, unfamiliar adult, small group – as well as in different contexts such as talking about things he has done, things he will do, things he is doing, things someone else is doing, and familiar and unfamiliar toys or activities. Finally, there are questions about the child's best and most frequent communicative situations.

The Pre-assessment Questionnaire is intended as a supplement to standard assessment procedures. It provides basic information about contextual factors influencing the child's communicative behaviors and is to be used prior to language sampling, so that more representative samples of the child's language may be obtained. Gallagher cites some examples of how useful this information can be in obtaining representative samples of children's language. One child had an MLU value of 1.6 in the clinician–child sample but an MLU of 3.96 when talking with her brother. One boy produced his most structurally complex utterances while playing with water toys in a plastic bucket filled with water, while for another it was when playing with a younger friend, and for yet another it was talking about pictures in a family album. An awareness of the influence of these contextual factors on performance also helps to clarify therapy goals by indicating the contexts in which the child appears to have greater difficulty.

The Pragmatics Profile of Early Communication Skills

This profile (Dewart and Summers, 1988) is also concerned with obtaining information about children's use of language in a variety of contexts, based on a questionnaire that is administered in an informal interview with parents or other caregivers.

The Pragmatics Profile is concerned with four aspects of the child's communication skills: communicative intentions, responses to communication, interaction and conversation, and contextual variation. Communicative intentions covers the range of speech acts a child uses, such as requesting, rejecting, protesting, greeting, naming, commenting, and giving information. Response to communication addresses questions such as how the parent gets the child's attention, how the child responds in interaction, whether the child understands gestures, acknowledges previous utterances, understands a speaker's intentions, and responds to "no", and occasions when the parent says things like "in a minute". Interaction and conversation include questions about interactive aspects of the child's communication, such as how exchanges are initiated and maintained, how the child initiates and responds to conversational repair, how the child terminates and joins conversations. The final aspect, contextual variation, examines the persons, places, times, and topics that produce the child's best communication, how the child uses language intrapersonally in play as well as interpersonally with peers, and the child's awareness of social conventions. Each category is illustrated with examples to help prompt the parent in providing information.

This profile is concerned with qualitative information about a child's communication skills. It is intended for use with infants and preschool children as a means of helping the clinician identify those aspects of the child's communication that need to be developed or modified, or where a further, more detailed investigation is warranted. There is a possible objection that parental reports may be unreliable as parents often do not know which aspects of the child's communication are important to report and which are not important. Moreover, parents may also either over-estimate or under-estimate their child's abilities because they are unaware of developmental norms. Against this the authors argue that parents know their children well and have wide experience of trying to communicate with them, so that information from the parents provides a useful guide to how the child communicates in everyday interactions outside the clinical situation.

Assessing the pragmatic ability of children
Roth and Spekman (1984) provide an organizational framework for the assessment of the pragmatic abilities of children. They divide communication skills into three levels of analysis: communicative intentions, presupposition, and the social organization of discourse. Communicative intention refers to the intended illocutionary acts that a child produces, such as requesting, naming, greeting, and responding. Two aspects of communicative intention are investigated: the range of different illocutionary acts used and understood by the child, and the child's ability to use and understand indirect as well as direct speech acts.

The term "presupposition" is used in a confusing way by Roth and Spekman. The usual definition within pragmatics was referred to in Chapter 2; this involved inferences or assumptions that are built into linguistic expressions (for example, that if someone *managed* to do something, this presupposes that they *tried* to do it). Roth and Spekman use the term "presupposition" to refer to the ability of children to make inferences about their conversational partner's knowledge. More usually, this ability is referred to as *role-taking*. The child's ability to make these inferences is reflected in the *content* and *form* of his or her messages – for example, the use of different styles for different communicative partners or for different physical contexts, such as face-to-face interaction as compared with telephone conversations.

The third level of assessment – social organization of discourse – deals with the ability to maintain a dialogue over several turns and includes conversational turn-taking, topic initiation, maintenance, termination, and shift as well as conversational repairs.

The main value of this framework is that it draws the attention of clinicians new to pragmatics to the major findings of the last 15 years or so. The main criticism of the framework is that it is not organized as a protocol with discrete, nonoverlapping, and well-motivated categories. Rather, a series of categories is presented based on comprehensive reviews of studies of pragmatic behavior in normally developing children. Terminological distinctions arising from differences in theoretical orientation are disregarded and there are no guidelines as to how the results of the analysis should be interpreted and translated into proposals for intervention.

An approach to developing conversational competence
Bedrosian (1985) presents a two-level approach to data analysis. His molecular level involves a fine-grained analysis of the child's behavior and

focuses primarily on topic. Each topic initiation is coded according to its subject matter, participant orientation (whether self-oriented or other-oriented), its communicative intent (as in Roth and Spekman, 1984), and whether eye contact is used for attention-getting. Subsequent turns are coded according to whether they are continuous or discontinuous for the discourse. Finally the interaction is coded according to the dimension of control, which is expressed by items such as interruptions and interrogatives. The second level of analysis, the molar analysis, is more global and is recommended for those observers operating under stricter time constraints. The molar level consists of a discourse skills checklist with sections for topic initiations, topic maintenance, use of eye contact, turn-taking, politeness, and some nonverbal behaviors. The categories in this checklist are simpler than those of Roth and Spekman (1984) and consist mainly of observational points such as: initiates new topics on a daily basis, talks mostly about self, responds to questions, interrupts others, uses commands, or uses nonverbal head nods to acknowledge. These are categorized by the observer.

As with the other checklists discussed earlier, Bedrosian's scheme covers a wide range of conversational behaviors and consists of categories that are largely self-explanatory. Furthermore, Bedrosian presents some useful ideas for improving deficient conversational skills. These consist of discourse goals and a series of teaching procedures which are clearly illustrated. So, for example, one goal might be to increase the child's frequency of topic initiations and the teaching procedures for this goal include practice in greetings, departures, ways of getting the listener's attention, expressing needs, making requests for information and for repair. While most of the discourse goals have the aim of increasing frequencies of behaviors, there is also a goal for decreasing the frequency of inappropriate topic initiations involving practice in items such as turn-taking, listening and decreasing interruptions. Thus the results of the checklist have to be interpreted by the observer according to their perceived appropriacy in order to determine what the discourse goal should be. This is perhaps the main weakness of this scheme, in that it leaves the most important part – the interpretation – to the observer's intuitions, although, to be fair, this weakness is shared by most other schemes and in any case it might be argued that most of the required interpretations can indeed be made by an insightful observer with sound commonsense. How this problem might be overcome will be discussed presently.

Towards a profile of conversational ability

The checklist presented in McTear (1985a) is similar to that of Roth and Spekman (1984), in that it is based on behaviors observed in normally developing children, although in McTear's checklist there is some attempt to motivate the categories in terms of a developmental sequence. The most basic category is turn-taking, which is a defining characteristic of conversation. Turn-taking precedes other pragmatic behaviors developmentally because it is possible for children to take turns in conversations before they have learned to fill out their turns with any meaningful linguistic content. Next comes the ability to produce contingently related turns. This involves as a minimum either the ability to initiate a conversational exchange, which includes getting the listener's attention and directing it to the objects and persons being referred to, or the ability to produce an appropriate response. At a more advanced level there are devices for introducing and re-introducing discourse topics and for drawing on background and shared knowledge (what Roth and Spekman (1984) describe as presupposition). Each of these skills can be seen in terms of its appropriacy, and in the case of this checklist requests for action are identified as a speech act whose appropriate usage requires a complex assessment of social considerations such as the role of the addressee and the nature of the requested task. Finally there is a section dealing with the main ways in which conversational breakdown can be repaired.

The main strength of McTear's scheme is that it presents a detailed summary of many of the key points of interest in developmental pragmatics, which is potentially useful in the analysis of disordered conversation. What is lacking, however, is a set of guidelines for the interpretation of results. Observers may quantify the frequencies of the many behaviors listed in the checklist but there is no suggestion as to how these frequencies are to be interpreted. Indeed, as seen later, it is not clear whether frequency is a useful index for conversational analysis in any case.

The Pragmatic Protocol

The Pragmatic Protocol (Prutting and Kirchner, 1987) is a descriptive taxonomy covering 30 pragmatic aspects of language. This protocol is designed mainly for use with children aged 5 years or older, although it has also proved useful as a means of providing an overall communicative index for adults (see the discussion of group comparison studies in Chapter 3). In this protocol each of the pragmatic skills falls under one of the following categories: verbal, paralinguistic, nonverbal. Verbal aspects include speech act pair analysis (taking speaker and listener roles appropriately), variety of speech acts, topic management (selection, introduction, maintenance, and change), and turn-taking, while paralinguistic aspects include intelligibility and fluency, and nonverbal aspects include physical proximity, body posture, and facial expressions. All of these items are coded according to whether they are used appropriately or inappropriately in the discourse.

The main strength of the Pragmatic Protocol is its comprehensiveness and its attempt to integrate verbal with paralinguistic and nonverbal behaviors. Each of the items is clearly defined and references are provided to indicate how the categories are motivated by the research literature. However, as with several other such taxonomies, there is no mention of how the different levels in the taxonomy relate to each other. Are some levels more general and others more specific? For example, is turn-taking initiation more specific than cohesion? Related to this, do some problems at one level predict problems at another level? For example, does a problem in topic maintenance affect turn-taking contingency?

Analysis of Language Impaired Children's Conversation – ALICC

ALICC (Adams and Bishop, 1989; Bishop and Adams, 1989) is based on the empirical studies involving group comparisons which were described in Chapter 3. The procedure consists of two parts: a quantitative analysis of aspects of children's conversational abilities and a detailed analysis of inappropriate language use.

The analysis of children's conversational abilities is based on the framework developed by McTear (1985a) and involves applying procedures developed for the analysis of normal conversational behavior to children with language impairment. The aspects that are examined are exchange structure, turn-taking, repairs, and cohesion. Exchange structure is concerned with different ways of initiating and responding in conversational sequences. Initiations are subdivided into questions, requests for action, and statements, while responses are coded as minimal or extended. The analysis of turn-taking is concerned with the identification of gaps and turn-taking violations. A distinction is made between inadvertent overlap, where the child has attempted to predict a turn completion point, and interruptions, in which turn-taking rules are violated (see the discussion of turn-taking in Chapter 4). Repairs include responses to requests for clarification – whether appropriate or inappropriate, the production of clarification requests, corrections of the other person's utterances, and self-repairs. Finally, cohesion focuses on the use of pronouns and demonstrative terms, distinguishing between cases where the pronoun either is recoverable from the linguistic context, the situation, or is ambiguous or unrecoverable.

Although these conversational features, when examined in the speech of language-impaired children, and especially those with pragmatic disability, can help to indicate the nature of the child's problems by indicating how the child's conversational behaviors differ from those of normal children, the authors argue that it is necessary also to examine the ways in which a child's language is inappropriate. The analysis of inappropriacy constitutes the second part of the procedure.

As a basis for the analysis of inappropriacy, transcripts of language-impaired and control children were examined and instances were identified of utterances where the normal flow of conversation appeared to be disrupted because the child's utterance was inappropriate in some way. These inappropriate utterances were then subcategorized as follows:

- *Expressive problems in syntax/semantics.* This category occurs where the child's utterance is inappropriate because of a linguistic problem – such as the wrong use of a lexical item (see the discussion of linguistic problems affecting pragmatic disability in Chapter 5 for some examples).
- *Failure to comprehend literal meaning.* This category includes cases where the child gives an inappropriate response to a question, which may have been due to misinterpretation or because the child only had a vague notion about what was being asked.
- *Pragmatic problems I: violation of exchange structure.* This category concerns failure to obey conversational sequencing rules, either by not responding at all or by ignoring the other person's initiation and continuing with an unrelated utterance.
- *Pragmatic problems II: failure to use context in comprehension.* The most typical example of this category is where a child responds to the literal meaning of a partner's utterance but misses its intended meaning – a meaning that can only be understood if the linguistic or situational context is taken into account, as in an indirect speech act.
- *Pragmatic problems III: too little information provided to partner.* In this case the child fails to provide information which the partner requires in order to make sense of an utterance, whether as a result of leaving out some important words on the wrong assumption that the listener has knowledge of them, the use of an unestablished referent, for example, by wrongly using a pronoun, or by omitting a logical step or crucial piece of information when telling a story or giving instructions.
- *Pragmatic problems IV: too much information provided to partner.* In this case the child over-elaborates on a topic saying more than is necessary to answer the question, repeats unnecessarily, or fails to use ellipsis appropriately.
- *Unusually or socially inappropriate content or style.* This category covers cases where the child goes off on a tangent and changes the topic inappropriately, fails to mark changes in topic, uses stereotyped language, asks questions to which the conversational partner could not possibly know the answer, or makes socially inappropriate remarks – for example, remarks that are over-friendly or over-personal.
- *Other problems.* This category covers examples where the child lacks knowledge or experience that is required for an adequate response.

All of these categories reflect aspects of pragmatic disability that have been reported in the literature and that were discussed extensively in Chapter 4. Bishop and Adams (1989) found that these categories could be used reliably to distinguish children with pragmatic disability from normal as well as from language-impaired children. They point out that many of the categories involve problems that are not specifically linguistic. For example, providing too much or too little information would appear to be a consequence of an inability to assess what the listener needs to know, while inappropriate questioning results from an inability to assess the listener's knowledge state. In both cases the problem is sociocognitive. However, when the child is unable to answer adequately owing to a lack of knowledge or experience, this reflects a cognitive disability.

Taken together, these two sets of measures can provide a profile of a child's conversational abilities and difficulties. The measure of conversational abilities is useful for providing a quantitative index when comparing subgroups of children or investigating how conversational competence varies in different settings. The analysis of inappropriacy provides a basis for a detailed investigation of specific areas of pragmatic difficulty and how these difficulties relate to the child's levels of linguistic, cognitive, and sociocognitive development. In this way this procedure addresses the issue of different types of pragmatic disability identified in Chapters 5 and 6 to a much greater extent than other checklists.

BLADES

BLADES (Bristol Language Development Scales, Gutfreund, Harrison and Wells, 1989) provides a comprehensive approach to the assessment of language production in children, involving the following areas: the purposes for which language is used in conversation (pragmatics), the meanings that are expressed (semantics), and the form and structure of the language used (syntax) (Gutfreund, Harrison and Wells, 1989). The first of these aspects is discussed in some detail.

The assessment of pragmatics in BLADES involves the analysis of the functions of utterances. Functions are defined as the purposes that utterances serve in conversation – to control the speech or actions of others (control function), exchange information (representative function), express feelings and attitudes or ask about the feelings and attitudes of others (expressive function), and to facilitate the channel of communication (procedural, social, and tutorial function). Each of these main functions is broken down into subfunctions. For example, control functions include requests for action, requests for permission, suggestions, statements of intention, offers. Each of these functions is assigned a level, based on the order of emergence of that function in a longitudinal study of a large group of children. Thus it is possible to compare the use of functions by a child and to determine whether the child's use of language is at average level for age. It is also possible to identify gaps in a child's functional use of language and to use the Therapy Planning Form, which sets out the functions according to type and level, to plan for the items that the child should learn next. The manual also includes detailed guidance as to the elicitation, transcription, and coding of utterances.

The potential value of BLADES becomes apparent when utterances are analysed at all three levels – pragmatics, semantics, and syntax – because it is then possible to determine links between a child's difficulties at these different levels. However, this cross-analysis of levels is not part of the procedure, although it would be possible to examine coded utterances to see which particular syntactic structures are used by a child to express a particular function, and, by comparing with samples from other children, to judge whether the child's range of structures for that function is restricted. As with similar schemes for coding the functions of utterances, there is the problem of identifying what function a particular utterance might have. The scheme allows for multiple coding of utterances. As an example: the utterance "I am going out now because it is raining" can be coded as both INTEND and GIVE EXPLANATION. This is a realistic approach, because clearly utterances may serve several functions simultaneously. However, there is the practical problem of knowing when to draw the line with multiple coding, because the coding scheme would permit utterances to be coded in many different ways and there is no way of deciding when the process is complete or whether some functions should be considered primary and others secondary. Obviously such considerations are important when it comes to making comparisons across samples. Notwithstanding these problems, the BLADES scheme provides a useful tool for the assessment of children's language production as a basis for diagnosis and therapy planning.

Some problems with checklists for pragmatics
As should be apparent from this brief review of checklists for pragmatics, all of these schemes cover roughly the same ground, with the main differences being in emphasis and grouping of items. This is hardly surprising, because the schemes have evolved out of extensive reviews of the developmental literature. The fact that there is this congruence and that the categories are well motivated is encouraging. However, there is still the problem that these categories may not be the most appropriate for pinpointing the types of problem that arise for language-impaired children. It may be the case that language-impaired children experience specific hurdles with certain aspects of language which are not specific hurdles for the normally developing child. For example, language-impaired children show marked problems with initiating conversations that are above and beyond what would be expected from normal controls of the same MLU (see the discussion of group design studies in Chapter 3).

For this reason case studies and ethnographic approaches will still be valuable. Furthermore, few of these checklists have been tested extensively with language-impaired subjects. A notable exception is the Prutting and Kirchner (1987) study discussed in Chapter 3 and it will be recalled that one of the main findings from this study was that there appeared to be different clusterings of pragmatic disabilities as well as wide variations within diagnostic groups. Bishop and Adams (1989) make a similar point.

The other main problem associated with checklists arises in their implementation. The simplest approach would seem to be to count frequencies of behaviors. However, the frequency or even the presence or absence of a behavior may not be the most important factor. Scores such as 80 percent do not make much sense and it is not even clear whether in some cases 80 percent is that much better than a score of 50 percent, because it may be the 20 percent that is deficient that has a devastating effect on communication. Indeed, in one case discussed by Prutting and Kirchner (1987), a single behavior, where a client entered the room and proceeded to lie down on the couch, had such a dramatic effect on the subsequent interaction even though it occurred only once.

Related to this is the question of the scoring method, in particular how judgments on appropriacy are made. Viewed abstractly by an outside observer, certain behaviors may appear inappropriate yet they may not have any adverse effect on the interaction. For this reason Prutting and Kirchner (1987) recommend the more conservative approach which only scores items as inappropriate if they have a perceived detrimental effect on the interaction. This allows for those cases where an individual produces compensatory strategies to further the interaction. What still cannot be accounted for, however, is the use of compensatory strategies by the person's conversational partner. It is possible to make someone's behaviors appear better than they might have been – the converse is also possible, of course – and the paradigm case of this is where mothers of very young infants make their babies appear to be more competent conversationalists than they really are by building conversations around whatever gestures or sounds they happen to produce (see the discussion of prelinguistic communication in Chapter 4). This is a paradox inherent in the study of interaction, which is, after all, *interpersonal* rather than *intrapersonal*, and for this reason any checklist which focuses on only one side of the interaction is bound to run into difficulty.

Standardized tests

From what has been said so far it might seem premature to think of standardized tests in the area of pragmatic disability as the field is so young and little is known about the range of disabilities that might fall under this general umbrella. However, it is also possible that the use of pragmatic tests in research might contribute to our understanding of pragmatic disability. Standardized tests have a further more practical value in that clinicians often require the support of such tests in demonstrating the need for a course of treatment for language disability, and until recently this was only possible in the more traditional areas of phonology, syntax and semantics. In this section a look is taken at one test for pragmatics which is in fairly wide use – the Test of Pragmatic Skills (Shulman, 1985).

Shulman's Test of Pragmatic Skills is intended for children suspected of having impairment in the appropriate use of conversational intentions or with a limited range of such intentions. Thus the focus is on the child's usage of illocutionary acts such as requesting information, requesting action, refusing and denying; and on their ability to choose an appropriate act in different communicative contexts. The main task for the tester is to elicit appropriate communicative intentions from the child in four standardized assessment tasks: playing with puppets, playing with a pencil and sheet of paper, playing with telephones, and playing with blocks. Some examples should make clear what is involved.

The puppet task involves two puppets, one of which the child is allowed to choose. Following this the clinician presents a series of probes that are intended to elicit a variety of illocutionary acts from the child including greeting, answering, informing, and naming. For example, the following are the probes for this task (for details of the other tasks, see Shulman, 1985):

1.   Let's talk! Hi!
2.   How are you today?
3.   I like to watch TV.
4.   Tell me what your favorite TV show is.
5.   I've never watched that show. Tell me about it.
6.   Do you know what my favorite show is?
7.   I like –_____ (clinician names a television show).
8.   Who are the good guys on your favorite TV show?
9.   Why are they good guys?
10. Thank you for talking with me. Bye-bye.

It should be fairly obvious what sorts of responses the child is required to make and in the test instructions sample responses and the illocutionary acts to be observed are set out for each probe. The child's response is scored on a six-point scale, as follows:

0   no response
1   contextually inappropriate
2   contextually appropriate nonverbal/gestural response only
3   contextually appropriate one-word response without elaboration
4   contextually appropriate response with minimal elaboration (two or three words)
5   contextually appropriate response with extensive elaboration (more than three words)

The child's total raw score on all four tasks is calculated and then divided by four to obtain the mean composite score (MCS) which is then used to determine the child's percentile rank. This is based on information obtained from a standardization sample of 650 children (see Shulman, 1985, for further details), which provides normative data across individual assessment tasks and mean composite scores.

The first point to note in the evaluation of this test is that it deals only with communicative intentions, which the author claims are an important foundation for functional communication. Communicative intentions are probably easier to elicit in standardized tests than other conversational behaviors, but even so, a wide range of responses could be predicted from even the fairly tightly constraining probes presented earlier, as the imaginative reader will no doubt have ascertained. This raises the question of scoring. Given that it is difficult to predict the full range of responses, rather too much has to be left to the tester in determining what score to assign. To take an example: one sample response to the probe "I've never watched that show. Tell me about it" is "I don't want to". This is described as rejection/denial but what score should be given? If the response is judged to be appropriate (and it is difficult to see why not), then should it receive maximum points on the grounds that it contains more than three words? How does this compare with a response that gives a long description of the show, which can only receive five points at a maximum? Indeed the child could go through most of the probes giving this type of response and score as well as a child who was more cooperative. In the same vein it can be argued that complexity is not necessarily a function of the length of an utterance and that a distinction between utterances of one word, two to three, and more than three words in length, is too simplistic.

A further problem relates to what scores from this test really tell us about a child's pragmatic abilities. Shulman puts forward the hypothesis that the scores might be used to predict young children's use of early discourse rules such as turn-taking, speaker dominance, topic maintenance and topic change, on the assumption that the child has demonstrated in the test the ability to express conversational intent. However, this hypothesis begs the question of the nature of the relationships between communicative intentions and these quite diverse discourse rules and it is possible to imagine children who might score well on this test but who still perform poorly in everyday conversations. In other words, the Test of Pragmatic Skills covers a restricted set of conversational behaviors, although it does provide a standardized and norm-referenced assessment instrument for measuring these behaviors. There is also a Language Sampling Supplement, covering turn-taking, speaker dominance, topic maintenance and topic change, which operates more or less along the lines of the checklists discussed earlier and which can be used to glean further information about the child's conversational abilities.

Pragmatic assessment: future prospects

The tools for pragmatic assessment that have been evaluated in this chapter have served the useful function of drawing the attention of clinicians to an important aspect of language which has until fairly recently been neglected in linguistics. However, this work must be seen as only the first stage in the development of realistic assessment instruments incorporating both the narrow and the broad views of pragmatics. Tests have the advantage that they can be quickly administered and can be standardized across a large sample to provide norm references, but they have the disadvantage that they focus on restricted aspects of language that are amenable to such testing. Checklists are more comprehensive, but they leave a lot to the clinician's intuitions in terms of making judgments about appropriateness as well as in interpreting the results. Ethnographic methods provide the most detailed analyses which permit individual and idiosyncratic profiles to emerge, but this method is too time-consuming for practicing clinicians, and for researchers there is the problem of comparability across studies.

Three problems have emerged from this discussion of pragmatic assessment. The first of these relates to the dimension of complexity. Many pragmatic functions can be accomplished in a variety of ways, all of which might be appropriate on a given occasion. Yet some of these devices will be more complex than others, either in terms of their linguistic or their conceptual complexity. Labelling items in terms of their illocutionary act function, such as request or denial, does not provide any information as to their complexity. At the moment judgments about complexity are made at a fairly intuitive level. There needs to be a more principled way of evaluating complexity in pragmatic categories (for one scheme which proposes a scale of conceptual complexity, see Blank and Franklin, 1980).

The second issue concerns the tendency to generalize from studies of normally developing children to a language-impaired population. As a first stage this strategy has been useful as a means of enumerating the factors that might be relevant. What is required now, however, is more research on language-impaired children in order to pinpoint those areas where problems tend to arise. If results were to emerge with any clarity this would result in less redundancy in assessment procedures because clinicians could focus on the most relevant categories within a more tightly constrained range.

Finally, there is a need to adopt, to a greater extent, the broad view of pragmatics and to integrate other aspects of language – phonologic, syntactic and semantic – with information on pragmatics. Most researchers pay lip service to this principle, advocating that scores from tests at other levels should be considered, but there needs to be more research on exactly how these different levels are to be integrated. For example, is a particular pragmatic deficit a consequence of a deficiency at some other level? Related to this is the question of how problems in pragmatics can be recast as deficits in conceptual and sociocognitive domains. For example, is the failure to take the listener's perspective a problem of language or of social cognition? The answer to questions such as this will determine the direction that therapy should take.

In this respect it might be useful to outline briefly the approach being used in an ongoing project at the Wolfson Centre in London (Allen, Jolleff and McConachie, 1990). This research is concerned with the assessment of children who seem to have problems with the semantic and pragmatic areas of language. More specifically, it had been noticed that several of the children in the study had similar behavior characteristics, such as obsessions and uncooperativeness, so that a major concern of the research was to investigate links between language and behavior in these children. Some examples are:

- using obsessions to make the world predictable when reasons for change or new events are hard to understand;
- becoming upset when told off, and not understanding why;
- becoming upset when unable to explain what they want, or why something is important.

To investigate these relationships between language and behavior, the investigators used a three-part assessment strategy:

- history taking, e.g. social interaction in the first year, reason for first referral, previous language assessments, previous cognitive assessments, current behavior such as attention span, nature of imaginative play, obsessions, home/school differences in behavior;
- standardized assessment, e.g. performance skills, reading, drawing, language tests.
- observation in unstructured and structured play situations.

This research is still in progress and the assessment strategy is still being developed. However, it illustrates the main points that have been made in this chapter and more generally throughout the book:

– it is important to gain a complete picture of the child's pragmatic abilities in different contexts;
– it is important to collect information that will enable us to consider relationships between the child's use of language and other potentially determining factors, such as (in this case) behavioral problems;
– in order to explain a child's pragmatic difficulties, it will be necessary to have information about earlier development and assessments, because the child's current difficulties may well be a consequence of earlier problems which themselves are no longer apparent.

In summary, there is a need for further work which takes into account both the narrow and the broad views of pragmatics, using a variety of methods, including longitudinal case studies and comparative samples, and integrating information from linguistic, social, and cognitive domains. This is an area where speech–language pathologists will be able to make a valuable contribution, both in the evaluation and improvement of currently available procedures and in the conduct of pragmatically oriented studies of language-impaired children. The present overview of assessment procedures should provide a guideline as to the tools that are currently available as well as indicating the sorts of assessment strategies that will prove most useful in future work.

Chapter 8
Future Directions

In this book the nature of pragmatic disability in children has been examined. First pragmatics was defined as an area of linguistics in which the main concern is with studying the use of language. Then approaches to language use were looked at in other disciplines which help us understand pragmatic disability. The main part of the book has been concerned with different aspects of pragmatic disability in children: how it has been studied; how pragmatic ability develops; the different ways in which children have difficulties with language use; relationships between pragmatic development and disability and linguistic, cognitive, sociocognitive, and affective development; and how pragmatic disability can be assessed.

In this chapter future directions are considered by examining two important issues in relation to pragmatic disability in children:

1. How to characterize it.
2. How to treat it.

Characterizing pragmatic disability

It has become clear in the course of the preceding chapters that the term "pragmatic disability" covers a wide range of impairments of language use and that the relationships between pragmatic disability and other impairments are complex. This has led us to suggest that there are different types of pragmatic disability. To recap: in some cases, children's use of language is affected by their limited linguistic knowledge – for example, a lack of the required structures or vocabulary. In other cases, children have difficulties with specific aspects of language use, despite having knowledge of the required structures. Other problems have even less to do with language – children may have difficulty in processing information; in assessing the requirements of their listeners; or they may have emotional problems that affect their ability to use language. These difficulties may

196

also be related to specific disabilities, such as mental handicap, learning disability, or autism. However, is there some way in which we can more accurately characterize pragmatic disability or should we simply accept the term as a convenient label for a range of difficulties that concern the use of language?

To answer this question, some interesting recent theoretical work on autism is considered. In Chapter 6 there was a review of Wing's proposal that autism should be seen in terms of a continuum of disorders that affect social interaction and that the main characteristics of this impairment of social interaction consist of a triad of common features involving: impairment of social recognition, impairment of social communication, and impairment of social imagination.

The recognition that autism is a disorder without clear boundaries and the proposal that a continuum best describes the characteristic disorder have led to the suggestion that pragmatic disability is just another term for autism (Aarons and Gittens, 1987; Wing, 1988). Similarly, the work of Weintraub and Mesulam (1982) on learning disabilities has also been suggested as representing higher levels in the autistic continuum. Indeed, if we take the major premise in Wing's argument as given, we could argue that it appears that the autistic continuum seems to extend itself to all pragmatic disabilities and also to specific disorders. For example, in Chapter 6 it was noted that some mentally handicapped, institutionalized persons appear socially inappropriate and disordered in their communicative interactions (Bredosian and Prutting, 1978; Prior et al., 1979) and it was also noted in the work of Donahue (1981) that learning-disabled children appear to be socially impaired. Are we then to say that all these children belong to the continuum of autism?

This strong position cannot be held. Wing (1988), in her discussion, of the autistic continuum, has attempted to draw on similarities in the style of communication in different disorders in an attempt to underline the importance and primacy of the triad. But, in putting this case forward, the argument has become circular, begging the question we ought to be asking – that is, what precisely might the relationships be between pragmatic abilities and other language and cognitive abilities? Do similarities in pragmatic problems point to similarities in the underlying reasons for the disorders?

Wing's approach has been one in which we take a clinically diagnosed syndrome such as autism, describe it fully, and use this description in the explanation of the disorder to provide a framework for understanding the disorder. The disadvantage of this approach is that it makes it difficult to compare similar behaviors across a range of clinically distinct etiologies without in some way reducing them to the original syndrome, autism.

One way forward has been provided by Bishop (1989) who argues that, although it is useful to draw attention to commonalities between disorders, it is important to consider more than one dimension in any continuum. Bishop discusses relationships between autism, pragmatic disability and a related impairment of social interaction called Asperger's syndrome. She suggests that two dimensions should be considered – that of interests and social relationships, as proposed by Wing (1988), and that of meaningful verbal communication. In this two-dimensional continuum categories are not distinct, they overlap and thus are best described by Venn diagrams, as shown in Figure 8.1. Autism would appear quite abnormal in the interests and social relationships axis and the behavior of individuals with autism would be variable in the meaningful verbal communication axis. Asperger's syndrome would overlap with autism and pragmatic disability but would be characterized by social relationships difficulties in conjunction with more normal meaningful verbal communication. Pragmatic disability would have more subtle abnormalities in both axes. It would also overlap with autism and Asperger's syndrome. In this way we acknowledge the presence of individuals who have the characteristics of the "core syndrome" but are also able to appreciate how these characteristics relate to the characteristics of other disorders. In addition, this approach allows us to understand those individuals who fall in the intersections between disorders. The model is attractive because in principle new axes or dimensions could be added to it as our knowledge of the disorders develops. Also, the present model is in line with current findings on research with autism and pragmatic disabilities carried out in the USA.

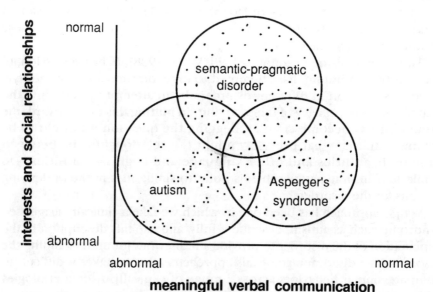

Figure 8.1 Two-dimensional model of the autistic continuum. (From Bishop, 1989, p. 117)

As mentioned in Chapter 3, Rapin and Allen (1983) coined the term "semantic–pragmatic disorders" to refer to children who are reasonably competent in phonology, grammar, and vocabulary but who have difficulty in language processing and language use. They identified a series of subtypes of language disorders based on *clinical* assessment of the child's phonologic, syntactic, semantic and pragmatic skills in spontaneous language during play (Rapin and Allen, 1983, 1986) supplemented with medical histories, neurologic examinations, and test results. Among the syndromes identified were word deafness (or verbal auditory agnosia), verbal dyspraxia, phonologic programming syndrome, phonologic–syntactic syndrome, lexical–syntactic syndrome and semantic–pragmatic syndrome (or, to use the terminology of this book, pragmatic disability). Thus, unlike the approach of Wing, the aim of these researchers was to subclassify developmental language disorders into finer categories because they suggested that language disorder was not a unitary diagnosis and that there did not appear to be a common element to all manifestations of language disorders.

Interestingly, these authors are carrying out a large study of children with dysphasia (language impairment) and autism in order to ascertain the prevalence of the different syndromes or types of disorder present in these two groups of children. A preliminary report of the findings was presented in Rapin and Allen (1987). In this report the first point is that a particular type or syndrome of language disorders is usually associated with clinically and etiologically very distinct groups of children, which suggests dysfunction in particular brain systems and not necessarily brain damage. Secondly, it was found that not all autistic children exhibited semantic–pragmatic disorders. Table 8.1 shows Rapin and Allen's (1987) classification of language-delayed and autistic children into the six subtypes. As can be seen from this table, only 28 percent of autistic children fell into the semantic–pragmatic category, suggesting that clinically recognized autistic children may vary in the language picture they present; and 7 percent of language-impaired children fell into the semantic–pragmatic category, suggesting that there are language-impaired children who experience problems in these areas but who are not clinically recognized as autistic.

Thus, it appears that the problem of classification is one which is ever evolving. Development arises both from a recognition of continuity among disorders and from discovery of distinctions within pre-existing categories (Bishop, 1989). Given our current state of knowledge these authors concur with Bishop in her treatment of the different diagnostic categories. First, in the interests of clarity of communication the term "autism" should be reserved for only those cases that fit the conventional diagnostic criteria suggested by Rutter (1978) and the American Psychiatric Association (1987). Secondly, where a child does not meet the

Table 8.1 Subclassification of language-impaired and autistic children by Rapin and Allen (1987)

Subtypes	Language impaired (%)	Autistic (%)
Verbal auditory agnosia	0	13
Verbal dyspraxia	14	0
Phonologic programming	21	2
Phonologic–syntactic	29	42
Lexical–syntactic	28	15
Semantic–pragmatic	7	28

criteria of autism and develops language age appropriately but with a mild to moderate form of the triad of social impairment, then a diagnosis of Asperger's syndrome should be considered. Bishop (1989) draws our attention to the fact that some psychiatrists use Asperger's syndrome more loosely to include any child of broadly normal intelligence with autistic features who nonetheless does not fit the conventional diagnostic criteria for autism. In this sense, Asperger's syndrome becomes one and the same with the American categorization of "pervasive developmental disorder not otherwise specified" (PDDNOS). Finally, Bishop argues that the term "specific semantic–pragmatic disorders" (pragmatic disability) be reserved for children who are not autistic in the conventional sense but who initially present with language delay and comprehension difficulties but continue to learn to talk clearly and grammatically. As these children develop, their pragmatic difficulties become more obvious. In this sense the picture for these children may be confusing at first, but as the child grows older the picture becomes clearer.

Another approach to the problem to pragmatic disabilities is exemplified by the work of McTear (1985a,b). As a linguist, McTear has argued that linguistics can provide a basis for describing different language disorders and pragmatic disabilities are no exception. This approach is based on the premise that classification and description of linguistic characteristics should proceed independently of other aspects of diagnosis. Thus, this approach has as its advantage the fact that comparisons can be made of similar disorders across a range of clinically distinct etiologies and that a detailed level of analysis of how the language system works can be provided and can complement attempts at subcategorization similar to those of Rapin and Allen (1983, 1987). The work of Crystal using this approach (Crystal, Fletcher and Garman, 1976; Crystal and Fletcher, 1979) has already proven most helpful in describing grammatical disability with the use of LARSP and it is recommended that this approach should be explored further. It is important that there is precise understanding of the possible relationships between the development of pragmatic abilities and of language abilities at other levels, as well as of how specific aspects of conversational interaction such as topic shifting and maintenance, turn-taking, appropriacy, and cohesion come together to form profiles of pragmatic disability.

Interestingly, this is already taking place. Bishop and her colleagues (Adams and Bishop, 1989; Bishop and Adams; 1989) have been carrying out research with pragmatic disorders funded by the Medical Research Council. Bishop has taken the linguistic approach in trying to identify and describe the key features of pragmatic disabilities in different groups of language-disordered children but she has gone a step further and found out whether there are specific features of the communicative system that differentiate one group of language-disordered children from another as well as from normal language learners. Bishop found that it was possible to develop a linguistically based procedure to describe pragmatic impairments that focused particularly on exchange structure, turn-taking, repair, cohesion, and inappropriacy. Her results, described in Chapter 3, are most interesting and provide us with much groundwork for future research.

Until recently, research on children with specific disorders has tended to compare the performance of disabled children to that of nondisabled children in a variety of situations and tasks. This search for "what is wrong" with disabled children has in some ways prevented us from understanding fully disabled children's behaviors in environmental and social terms (Ryan, 1975; Leudar, 1981; Beveridge, 1989). The situations and tasks under which mentally handicapped, learning-disabled and autistic children have been studied have sometimes been quite arbitrary in the sense that they do not provide us with information about social factors which influence their daily lives. This approach has seen a major shift with the pragmatic revolution and the awareness of social–cognition and ecological considerations in research. This is not to say that carefully controlled, comparative studies are not important, but that we need to supplement this type of research design by studying the interactions between disabled persons and key people in their lives. It is our hope that the different perspectives discussed here may allow us to understand how the social–communicative system works for the individual as well as how it compares with the norm.

Treating pragmatic disability

We have experienced almost three decades, since the early 1960s, away from the traditional medical service models which dichotomized diagnostic from treatment functions. Speech–language pathologists have long been active in the integration of assessment and intervention, and in theory and in practice have treated them as two sides of the same coin (Muma, 1978; Launer and Lahey, 1981). We believe this amalgamation of identification and management of language problems is essential for appropriate intervention with disordered children, and the separation of assessment and remediation into different chapters in this book is done solely for the purposes of exposition. As we shall see, the same issues that were raised in assessment are pertinent to intervention procedures. It is necessary to consider the general impact of pragmatics on intervention as well as how to remediate pragmatic difficulties. First, the impact of the current pragmatic framework on intervention is considered, followed by a focus on the resources available to us to remediate pragmatic disorders.

The pragmatic revolution

The pragmatic approach has emphasized the interactional nature of language assessment and remediation. As discussed in Chapter 3, a broad view of pragmatics affects all aspects of our involvement with children because it becomes clear that all language is pragmatically based and that it is the social use of language that gives rise to structure and content (Cole, 1982; Gallagher and Prutting, 1983).

With this in mind it is necessary to reconceptualize goals and procedures. Craig (1983) provides us with the foundations to do this. For intervention goals, the pragmatic framework brings communicative aims to the centerpoint making them the most basic steps in intervention planning. It is no longer acceptable to leave generalization as a final stage in the intervention process where what has been taught will be used by the child in everyday conversation. Everyday, natural communication is the aim from the start whether our interest lies in advancing the child's use of syntax or in helping the child to become a more active participant in conversation. The amalgamation of the conversational–social nature of the situation with the structural–linguistic knowledge necessary to participate in it becomes the first priority for speech–language pathology goal-setting. The actual goals have also been enriched. Not only are we remediating problems with structure and content but also problems with language use in social interaction. Some language-impaired children appear to have difficulties with the pragmatic aspects of language independent of their structural knowledge of the language (Conti-Ramsden and Friel-Patti, 1983,1984) and further still some children appear to have as their major problem language use (Rapin and Allen, 1983; McTear, 1985b; Conti-Ramsden and Gunn, 1986; Bishop and Rosenbloom, 1987). As Snow et al. (1984) suggested, this means that our clinical goals now focus on phonology, syntax, semantics, as well as pragmatics (pragmatics in the narrow sense discussed in Chapters 1 and 3) and that no matter what area is focused on, the goals have to be communicative in that they will create or take advantage of natural contexts where partners share a topic of interest, where turn-taking is shared, and where meaning is continually negotiated, in other words, where the concept of broad pragmatics is put into effect.

Craig (1983) also points to the need to reconceptualize our procedures in the light of the pragmatic revolution. Pragmatics underlines the importance of individual differences across children and interactional style differences across situations and conversational partners. In this approach it is the process that is essential not the product, because conversation and interaction themselves are seen as the context in which language learning occurs (Waterson and Snow, 1978; Wells, 1981; Snow et al., 1984). Through interaction with others and in different situations, the child learns to develop his or her communicative system in order to achieve successful communication.

More specifically, different researchers have suggested various ways in which intervention procedures need to change in order to take into account the paradigm shift towards a pragmatic framework. Snow et al. (1984) argue that our procedures need to include communicatively useful language, semantically contingent language, and language that fosters the negotiation of meaning. The importance of communicatively useful language should be emphasized. The clinician needs to use language in intervention that will enable the child to become a participant in the conversation. The more useful the language is to the child, the more valuable it becomes in intervention. Snow points out that this forces the clinician to investigate the language environments of the child. Thus a child enrolled in preschool needs language relating to playground equipment, snacks, possessions, while a child who is at home all the time may find, for example, language relating to requesting favorite activities and foods more useful. As discussed in Chapter 5, the child's acquisition of language is facilitated when adults follow the child's topic and incorporate into their utterances the focus of the preceding utterance by the child. This implies that in remediation the clinician follows the child's lead and builds on it to provide the necessary language models for language growth. Thus, if the child chooses a book to read, both clinician and child could engage in conversation about the content of the book, turning pages, opening and closing the book – all communicatively useful language in the book-reading context. Finally, meaning can be negotiated through requests for clarification which serve the important function of continuing the child's topic but indicating to the child that the message was not clear and that it needs to be revised if successful communication is to be achieved.

In the same vein, Craig (1983) and Muma (1978, 1983) have suggested that pragmatics has turned the three most important points in the clinicians' agenda for organizing intervention into questions. Not so long ago, intervention was delivered by the clinician according to a plan of what the clinician and the child should say. Now these same points are questions:

– Who should the intervention agents be?
– What should the intervention agents say and do in the remediation interaction?
– What is the child expected to do and say in the remediation interaction?

The first of these questions is addressed by reviewing briefly research on the nature of clinician–child interaction.

Clinician–child interaction

Our understanding that communicative competence develops within the context of social interaction implies that the clinician cannot be the sole intervention agent in remediation. Children vary their language use as a function of the characteristics of the conversational partner; thus children need to experience this in order to become effective communicators. Thus, peer interaction, parent–child interaction, caregiver–child interaction and teacher–child interactions are all contexts in which the conversational partner can act as an intervention agent. However, the speech–language pathologist still plays a central role in remediation. Speech–language pathologists, with their training and expertise, are able to provide the child with increased experience of success in communicative interaction. It is in interaction with the clinician that the child gets equipped with the necessary tools to communicate and it is with the clinician as consultant that the interaction with others should take place. For this reason, it is useful to examine research that has investigated the ways in which clinicians and children interact.

There is a dearth of research in this area and what has been published appears to be outdated given current clinical practice in speech–language pathology. Thus, Prutting et al. (1978) used various pragmatic procedures to analyze clinician–child discourse in a language-remediation setting. They found that the most prominent pattern of interaction was for clinicians to request and for the children to respond to requests. McTear (1985a) also found a similar pattern in his observations. Furthermore, clinicians most often requested verbal information or requested *yes/no* answers. For example:

(Clinician holds a picture of a boy riding a tricycle)
T: What is the boy doing?

(Clinician holds a picture of a dog under a chair)
T: Is the dog on the chair?

Prutting rightly points out that the communicative function of these questions is not evident given that both the speaker and the listener know the information being requested. The questions were actually used as a technic to elicit specific syntactic structures which resulted in language being remediated outside the need to communicate. In their data they also found that the most common request for qualification by the clinician was a request to provide a more complete answer. For example:

(Clinician holds a picture of a man wearing a hat)
T: What is the man wearing?
C: A hat
T: Say the whole thing
C: The man is wearing a hat
T: Good

The researchers once again point out that elliptical responses to wh-questions are conversationally more appropriate than the complete sentences and thus they question the value of eliciting a particular syntactic structure in a context that is not appropriate in natural conversation. McTear discusses one other pattern in clinician–child interaction. The following is the example he uses (McTear, 1985a, p. 256):

(Looking at some pictures together)
T: Let's have a look at some pictures
        What's this one about?
C: Milk
T: What time is it at school?
C: Break-time
T: And what are the children doing?
C: Drinking milk
T: That's right
        Why are there some empty bottles in the crate?
C: Drink all
T: That's right
        Those children have drunk it all up

McTear suggests that the predominant discourse pattern of clinician–child interaction is that of initiation by the clinician, response by the child and maybe feedback from the clinician. Furthermore, the clinician seems continually to be moving on to a new focus in the topic once that exchange of initiation, response and possible feedback has been finished. Work by

Spinelli and Ripich (1985) and Letts (1985) further supports this finding with the important proviso that there are large individual differences in the extent to which this pattern is used by clinicians.

Letts (1985, 1989) suggests that on average the pattern of clinician as initiator and child as responder occurs approximately two-thirds of the time, but individual variation makes it impossible to make generalizations. Furthermore, Letts continues to do a finer-grained analysis of the communicative acts used by speech–language pathology in order to examine further the patterns of interaction exhibited in therapy. She found two types of communicative acts used by clinicians: organizing acts and ongoing acts. Organizing acts set the therapy activity in motion and they ensure that the activity does not break down. Thus, attention-getters, boundary markers, requests for clarification are all considered as organizing acts. Testing questions, directives, feedback, and others are considered as ongoing acts. Letts found that 90 percent of all acts used in therapy fell into the above categories. The remaining 10 percent consist of social acts, such as greetings and goodbyes. Interestingly, all clinicians used organizing acts between 8 percent and 15 percent of the time. What was less consistent was the use of ongoing acts. Clinicians varied greatly as to what type of ongoing act they used to elicit a response from the client and the extent to which they used the different types of ongoing acts.

Using another approach to the analysis of clinician–client interaction, Hansson and Nettelbladt (1990) found that in Sweden, clinician–client interactions also had the structure of clinician as initiator and child as responder. Of particular interest, however, was their finding that clinicians' interaction style changed as the language-impaired children developed. Clinicians take the initiator role less often as the child's syntax develops and, conversely, the child takes the initiator role more often and provides more expanded responses once his or her grammar develops. This finding, taken together with the more recent work on individual differences in speech–language pathology interaction, points a way forward for research. As mentioned at the outset practicing clinicians are definitely aware of the criticisms and problems identified in clinician–client interaction. In addition, clinicians do not consider that the data gathered a few years ago are representative of therapeutic practice today. Further research is needed to learn and evaluate how clinician–child interactions currently work within the framework of individual differences and changes in development. This is an area where research coming from clinicians themselves would be invaluable.

Pragmatic issues in intervention

Earlier questions were raised about what the intervention agents were and what the child should do and say in intervention situations. These two questions can be addressed simultaneously. The pragmatic perspective brings more symmetry between the intervention agents and the child in communication than was previously assumed in other procedures. Conversational interaction is the center and main focus of the intervention sequence and thus remediation procedures can be based on varying the content, pace and sequencing of conversations as long as the interaction remains natural and meaningful. Thus, for the young child, play continues to be a favorite activity within pragmatic approaches because play provides a natural context in which child and intervention agents can engage in meaningful conversational interaction. The child can choose the focus of attention by choosing a toy to play with and conversation can develop from this initial point. This does not mean that play or any type of interaction in remediation should be totally unplanned in order for it to be meaningful and natural. The clinician can plan and organize the child's communicative experiences to maximize the opportunities for the child to encounter what the child needs to learn. Thus, at snack time in a language unit the clinician and teacher leave out a child when handing biscuits, creating a context in which a request of some sort is appropriate (for further speech–language pathology ideas see Constable 1983, 1986; Winitz, 1983; Wiig and Semel, 1984; Fey, 1986; Beveridge and Conti-Ramsden, 1987). As the child grows older, clinicians should look at the child's environment to derive remediation interactions that are meaningful and interesting for the child. Thus the older child may enjoy rule-governed games, role-play, and active discussions on particular topics such as a favorite TV show.

The above discussion provides us with ideas for pragmatic intervention. As mentioned pragmatic considerations permeate all aspects of intervention with all types of children. In addition, however, it is necessary to consider further the group of children who appear to have specific problems with language use whether they appear to have other problems with language such as the specific language-disordered children studied by Conti-Ramsden (Conti-Ramsden and Friel-Patti, 1983; 1984) or they appear to have little difficulty with structural aspects of language such as pragmatically disordered children (Rapin and Allen, 1983; McTear, 1985b). The development of intervention approaches to help these children overcome their pragmatic difficulties is only just beginning and research as to their efficacy is most needed. In the next section various therapeutic approaches are discussed which may prove useful in the treatment of children with pragmatic disabilities. This section is offered tentatively as a starting point from which clinical evaluation and research can take place.

Intervention and pragmatic disabilities

It will sound repetitive to say that all intervention procedures for pragmatically disabled children need also to fall within the guidelines for pragmatic intervention outlined above. This interplay between a broad and narrow view of pragmatics needs to be clear in our minds so that it does not become a source of confusion in assessment and intervention. When the speech–language pathology goal is to help the child learn the rules of social–conversational interaction it may be found that some approaches lend themselves more than others for this purpose. As mentioned before, these are suggestions and we must await research before any firm conclusions can be drawn.

With young children *play* is considered to be one of the most fertile grounds for intervention. Conti-Ramsden and Gunn (1986) used play in intervention with Tony, a child with pragmatic disability. They found that in the play situation the clinician, teacher and other children modelled early interactional skills such as turn-taking and eye contact. Modelling involves using a verbal or nonverbal behavior in the appropriate context which the child can observe, but is not required to imitate or to produce the behavior. The child is thus left to pick up the model and transfer it to his communicative system. In the play context, it appears that explicit verbal coaching also occurs and this procedure has been found to produce changes in the social interaction of socially isolated normal language learners (Oden and Asher, 1977; Craig, 1983) and has been observed to occur in parent–child talk especially with respect to teaching politeness, for example, "Can you say thank you?" (Becker, 1990). Its effect with language-disordered children has yet to be evaluated but this technique appears promising. *Explicit verbal coaching* involves stating conversational principles to the child and this often occurs naturally in peer interaction with young children. Craig offers the example of a 3-year-old boy who while playing said to a child client who had difficulty verbally turn-taking: "No, no. I am going to speak to you and then you speak back."

More recently, Norris and Damico (1990) have also suggested that children should be allowed to explore and experience language. They argue that language learning is not, and should not be, "correct" or error-free, because the child can learn from errors. Adult's verbal coaching can play a role in fostering advances and making children realize the state of their current communicative system.

Beveridge and Conti-Ramsden (1987, Chapter 7) also describe the use of explicit verbal coaching with an older pragmatically disabled 11-year-old child. Their use of verbal coaching was done in the context of role-play. Social role enactment or role-play has been an area of much study in the normal development literature and it is necessary to apply and evaluate this information further for use in intervention (Mann and Mann, 1966; Sachs and Devin, 1976; Rubin, 1980; Fein, 1981; Watson, 1981). In role-play routine interactions such as going shopping, borrowing something from a peer, talking on the telephone are enacted, each person taking a role, such as customer or shop owner, with all the props necessary to set up a real-life situation. In Beveridge and Conti-Ramsden (1987) the client child was involved with the teacher and peers in role-play, and the clinician accompanied the child and coached him through the interaction, for example, telling him he needed to greet the shop owner, to thank the person from whom you borrowed something, to say good bye once he finished talking on the phone. The clinician and teacher also devised a communication copybook which containing explicit verbal coaching in writing. All the essential steps involved in a particular interaction such as borrowing something were identified, talked about, and sequentially written down. Then the child could look through the copybook in the way an actor would look through his or her cue cards before the child would go through with the interaction. Indeed the whole area of drama and the arts needs to be studied for its intervention potential with language-disordered children (Hutt, 1986).

Beveridge and Tatham (1976) found that mentally handicapped children and adolescents improved with experience of *referential communication tasks*. In their study, the less able adolescents learned from the more able adolescents and they concluded that referential tasks may facilitate the development of conversation. Referential communication tasks involve two people who are usually separated by a screen of some sort, so one person cannot see what the other person has or does but they can hear each other. One person has to tell the other about something or how to do something. The task can vary. Thus, one subject may be asked to describe a picture to the other person, or give the other person instructions as to what object or card needs to be picked up or needed etc. The task and set-up need not be stilted and can involve games that interest the child or adolescent. McTear (1985a, Chapter 9) also used referential communication tasks when assessing the abilities of a child with pragmatic disability. He found that the child in question failed as speaker to take the listener's perspective and often underspecified the information for the listener. Research in this area, like that carried out by Beveridge and Tatham (1976), is needed to see if children with pragmatic disabilities improve with experience of referential communication tasks.

Another interesting approach has been outlined by Smedley (1989). Smedley suggests that children with pragmatic disabilities can benefit from having written work that complements their oral language pathology. The activities suggested require a reading age of 6;6 years. Smedley found that 85 percent of the children with pragmatic disabilities whom he encountered were able to participate and benefit from this approach. The following example illustrates the nature of the activities suggested.

Smedley argues that children with pragmatic disabilities have particular difficulties with temporality – that is, tense selection, ordering events within a narrative, and using time vocabulary. But, because spatial concepts are acquired by children before temporal concepts, Smedley argues that spatial concepts need to be looked at and worked on first. He suggests working with practical demonstrations as well as using cloze procedures and pictures which can be backed up with manual sign systems such as Paget–Gorman. Exercises with "before" and "after" such as "I wake up _____ I get up" or "I go into the classroom _____ I sit at my desk" are illustrated as well as other activities that are worth exploring.

Another possibly useful area discussed by McTear (1985a) is *social skills training*. Social skills training is concerned with how the skills of face-to-face interaction may be improved. This area grew from a practical concern such as how to teach adolescents to improve their job interview techniques, or how a counselor or social worker should help persons in need to engage in interaction (Hargie, Saunders and Dickson, 1987). The procedure is simple and not novel. First, the skills relevant to the needs of the trainee are identified, for example, questioning, reflection and reinforcement for the counselor. Then, these skills are talked about, taught and practiced usually in role-play situations which are video recorded and then analyzed (see Rustin and Kuhr, 1989, for suggestions for social skills activities). McTear (1985a) has suggested that social skills training could be useful in helping children with pragmatic disabilities but the approach needs to be complemented with a more in-depth consideration of issues such as the identification of skills, the description of linguistic behavior, and the dynamic, reciprocal nature of interaction – all areas in which linguistics and particularly pragmatics have a major role to play. Once again we need research and clinical practice to suggest guidelines for the application of different approaches to the remediation of pragmatic disabilities.

Concluding remarks

In this chapter some directions have been suggested for future work in the area of pragmatic disability in children. First some recent theoretical work on autism was reviewed – in particular, on the continuum of autistic disorders – which has been used to characterize and explain pragmatic disability. It was suggested, however, that this approach fails to account for some of the types of pragmatic disability that have been described in this book. For this reason an approach is recommended in which the key features of a child's pragmatic difficulties are identified and classified, and these are examined in relation to other information about the child. It is only after such careful examination that explanatory statements about the determining factors of the pragmatic difficulties should be stated.

The second main point in this chapter concerned the treatment of pragmatic disability. Assuming that the child's difficulties have been carefully identified in the light of the recommendations given, the pragmatic perspective indicates a more interactionally based approach to intervention. Some useful procedures were outlined that fall within this perspective, although it was also indicated that further research is necessary to validate the efficacy of these procedures.

Pragmatic disability is a complex phenomenon. An attempt has been made in this book to clarify for researchers and practitioners the most important questions to address. These research questions are interesting in themselves and should continue to tax our minds for some time to come. The important contribution that practicing clinicians can make to this process is also stressed because they are in regular contact as professionals with children who have difficulty in using language to communicate. However, the most important consideration should be that our greater understanding of the nature and causes of pragmatic disability should ultimately enhance the quality of life for those children unfortunate enough to be impaired in this way.

References

Aarons, M. and Gittens, T. (1987) *Is this Autism?* Windsor, Berkshire: NFER-Nelson

Abbeduto, L. and Rosenberg, S. (1980) The communicative competence of mildly retarded adults. *Applied Psycholinguistics* **1**, 405–426

Abbeduto, L. and Rosenberg, S. (1985) Children's knowledge of the presuppositions of "know" and other cognitive verbs. *Journal of Child Language* **12**, 621–641

Abbeduto, L. and Rosenberg, S. (1987) Linguistic communication and mental retardation. In S.Rosenberg (ed.) *Advances in Applied Psycholinguistics, Vol. 1: Disorders of First Language Development*. Cambridge: Cambridge University Press

Ackerman, B.P. (1978) Children's understanding of speech acts in unconventional directive frames. *Child Development* **49**, 311–318

Adams, C. and Bishop, D.V.M. (1989) Conversational characteristics of children with semantic-pragmatic disorder. I. Exchange structure, turntaking, repairs and cohesion. *British Journal of Disorders of Communication* **24**, 211–239

Adams, J.L. and Ramey, C.T. (1980) Structural aspects of maternal speech to infants reared in poverty. *Child Development* **51**, 1280–1284

Allen, J., Jolleff, N. and McConachie, H. (1990) Semantic-pragmatic disorder: behaviour language links. Paper presented at First Workshop on Semantic-Pragmatic Disorders, Wolfson College, London, January 1990

American Psychiatric Association (1987) *Diagnostic and Statistical Manual,* 3rd edn, Revised (DSM-III-R). Washington, DC: American Psychiatric Association

Anselmi, D., Tomasello, M. and Acunzo, M. (1986) Young children's responses to neutral and specific contingent queries. *Journal of Child Language* **13**, 135–144

Astington, J.W. (1988) Children's production of commissive speech acts. *Journal of Child Language* **15**, 411–423

Astington, J.W. (1990) Metapragmatics: children's conception of promising. In G.Conti-Ramsden and C.E.Snow (eds) *Children's Language, Vol. 7*. Hillsdale, NJ: Erlbaum

Astington, J.W., Harris, P.L. and Olson, D.R. (eds)(1988) *Developing Theories of Mind*. Cambridge: Cambridge University Press

Atkinson, J.M. and Drew, P. (1979) *Order in Court*. London: Macmillan

Atkinson, M. (1979) Prerequisites for reference. In E. Ochs and B. Schieffelin (eds) *Developmental Pragmatics*. New York: Academic Press

Attwood, A., Frith, U. and Hermelin, B. (1988) The understanding and use of interpersonal gestures by autistic and Down's syndrome children. *Journal of Autism and Developmental Disorders* **18**, 241–257

Baker, L. and Cantwell, D.P. (1982) Psychiatric disorder in children with different types of communication disorders. *Journal of Communication Disorders* **15**, 113–126

Baker, N. and Nelson, K.E. (1984) Recasting and related conversational techniques for triggering syntactic advances in young children. *First Language* **5**, 3–22

Baltaxe, C.A.M. (1977) Pragmatic deficits in the language of autistic adolescents. *Journal of Pediatric Psychology* **2**, 176–180

Baltaxe, C.A.M. and Simmons, J.Q. (1977) Language patterns of adolescent autistics: a comparison between English and German. In P.Mittler (ed.) *Research to Practice in Mental Retardation*, Vol. II: *Education and Training*. Baltimore: University Park Press

Baltaxe, C.A.M. and Simmons, J.Q. (1988) Pragmatic deficits in emotionally disturbed children and adolescents. In R. Schiefelbusch and L. Lloyd (eds) *Language Perspectives*, 2nd edn. Austin, Texas: Pro-Ed

Barbieri, M.S., Colavita, F. and Scheuer, N. (1990) The beginning of the explaining capacity. In G.Conti-Ramsden and C.E. Snow (eds) *Children's Language*, Vol. 7. Hillsdale, NJ: Lawrence Erlbaum

Barnes, S., Gutfreund, M., Satterly, D. and Wells, G. (1983) Characteristics of adult speech which predict children's language development. *Journal of Child Language* **10**, 665–684

Baron-Cohen, S. (1987) Autism and symbolic play. *British Journal of Developmental Psychology* **5**, 139–148

Baron-Cohen, S. (1988) Social and pragmatic deficits in autism: cognitive or affective? *Journal of Autism and Developmental Disorders* **18**, 379–402

Baron-Cohen, S. (1989a) The autistic child's theory of mind: a case of specific developmental delay. *Journal of Child Psychology and Psychiatry* **30**, 285–298

Baron-Cohen, S. (1989b) Are autistic children behaviourists? An examination of their mental-physical and appearance-reality distinctions. *Journal of Autism and Developmental Disorders* **19**, 579–600

Baron-Cohen, S. (1989c) Do autistic children have obsessions and compulsions? *British Journal of Clinical Psychology* **28**, 193–200

Baron-Cohen, S., Leslie, A.M. and Frith, U. (1985) Does the autistic child have a "theory of mind"? *Cognition* **21**, 37–46

Baroni, M.R. and Axia, G. (1989) Children's meta-pragmatic abilities and the identification of polite and impolite requests. *First Language* **9**, 285–297

Bates, E. (1976) *Language and Context*. New York: Academic Press

Bates, E. (1979) *The Emergence of Symbols*. New York: Academic Press

Bates, E., Camaioni, L. and Volterra, V. (1975) The acquisition of performatives prior to speech. *Merrill-Palmer Quarterly* **21**, 205–226

Bates, E. and MacWhinney, B. (1982) Functionalist approaches to grammar. In E. Wanner and L. Gleitman (eds) *Language Acquisition: The State of the Art*. Cambridge: Cambridge University Press

Bateson, M.C. (1975) Mother-infant exchanges: the epigenesis of conversational interaction. In D. Aaronson and R.W. Rieber (eds) *Developmental Psycholinguistics and Communicative Disorders. Annals of the New York Academy of Science* **263**, 101–112

Bateson, M.C. (1979) The epigenesis of conversational interaction: a personal account of research development. In M. Bullowa (ed.) *Before Speech: The Beginning of Interpersonal Communication*. Cambridge: Cambridge University Press

Beal, C. and Flavell, J.H. (1981) Comprehension in a referential communication task. *Child Development* **54**, 148–153

Becker, J.A. (1982) Children's strategic use of requests to mark and manipulate social status. In S.Kuczaj (ed.) *Language Development*, Vol.. 2: *Language, Thought, and Culture*. New York: Springer

Becker, J.A. (1990) Processes in the acquisition of pragmatic competence. In G.Conti-Ramsden and C.E. Snow (eds) *Children's Language*, Vol. 7. Hillsdale, NJ: Lawrence Erlbaum

Bedrosian, J.L. (1985) An approach to developing conversational competence. In D.N. Ripich and F.M. Spinelli (eds) *School Discourse Problems*. San Diego: Singular Publishing Group

Bedrosian, J.L. and Prutting, C.A. (1978) Communicative performance of mentally retarded adults in four conversational settings. *Journal of Speech and Hearing Research* **21**, 79–95

Bernard-Opitz, V. (1982) Pragmatic analysis of the communicative behavior of an autistic child. *Journal of Speech and Hearing Disorders* **47**, 99–109

Beveridge, M. (1989) Social cognition and the communicative environment of the mentally handicapped. In M. Beveridge, G. Conti-Ramsden and I.Leudar (eds) *Language and Communication in Mentally Handicapped People*. London: Routledge, Chapman & Hall

Beveridge, M. and Conti-Ramsden, G. (1987) *Children with Language Disabilities*. Milton Keynes: Open University Press

Beveridge, M. and Evans, P. (1978) Classroom interaction: two studies of severely subnormal children. *Research in Education* **19**, 39–48

Beveridge, M. and Hurrell, P. (1980) Teachers' responses to the initiations of ESN(S) children. *Journal of Child Psychology and Psychiatry* **21**, 175–182

Beveridge, M., Spencer, J. and Mittler, P. (1979) Self-blame and communication failure in retarded adolescents. *Journal of Child Psychology and Psychiatry* **20**, 129–138

Beveridge, M. and Tatham, A. (1976) Communication in retarded adolescents: utilization of known language skills. *American Journal of Mental Deficiency* **81**, 96–99

Bilmes, J. (1988) The concept of preference in conversation analysis. *Language in Society* **17**, 161–181

Bishop, D.V.M. (1989) Autism, Asperger's syndrome and semantic-pragmatic disorder: where are the boundaries? *British Journal of Disorders of Communication* **24**, 107–122

Bishop, D.V.M. and Adams, C. (1989) Conversational characteristics of children with semantic-pragmatic disorder. II. What features lead to a judgement of inappropriacy? *British Journal of Disorders of Communication* **24**, 241–263

Bishop, D. and Rosenbloom, L. (1987) Classification of childhood language disorders. In W. Yule and M. Rutter (eds) *Language Development and Disorders*. Oxford: MacKeith Press

Blank, M. and Franklin, E. (1980) Dialogue with preschoolers: a cognitively-based system of assessment. *Applied Psycholinguistics* **1**, 127–150

Blank, M., Gessner, M. and Esposito, A. (1979) Language without communication: a case study. *Journal of Child Language* **6**, 329–352

Bliss, L.S. (1985) The development of persuasive strategies by mentally retarded children. *Applied Research in Mental Retardation* **6**, 437–447

Bloom, L. and Lahey, M. (1978) *Language Development and Language Disorders*. New York: Wiley

Bloom, L., Rocissano, L. and Hood, L. (1976) Adult-child discourse: developmental interaction between information processing and linguistic knowledge. *Cognitive Psychology* **8**, 521–552

Bondurant, J.L., Romeo, D.J. and Kreschmer, R. (1983) Language behaviors of mothers of children with normal and delayed language. *Language, Speech and Hearing Services in Schools* 14, 233–242

Borys, S.V. (1979) Factors influencing the interrogative strategies of mentally retarded and nonretarded students. *American Journal of Mental Deficiency* 84, 280–288

Boucher, J. (1989) The theory of mind hypothesis of autism: explanation, evidence and assessment. *British Journal of Disorders of Communication* 24, 181–198

Bransford, J.D. and McCarrell, N.S. (1974) A sketch of a cognitive approach to comprehension: some thoughts about understanding what it means to comprehend. In W.B. Weimer and D.S. Palermo (eds) *Cognition and the Symbolic Processes*. Hillsdale, NJ: Lawrence Erlbaum

Bredart, S. (1984) Children's interpretation of referential ambiguities and pragmatic inference. *Journal of Child Language* 11, 665–672

Bretherton, I. and Beeghly-Smith, M. (1982) Talking about internal states: the acquisition of an explicit theory of mind. *Developmental Psychology* 18, 906–921

Brinton, B. and Fujiki, M. (1982) A comparison of request-response sequences in the discourse of normal and language-disordered children. *Journal of Speech and Hearing Disorders* 47, 57–62

Brinton, B., Fujiki, M. and Sonnenberg, E.A. (1988) Responses to requests for clarification by linguistically normal and language-impaired children in conversation. *Journal of Speech and Hearing Disorders* 53, 383–391

Brinton, B., Fujiki, M., Loeb, D.F. and Winkler, E. (1986) Development of conversational repair strategies in response to requests for clarification. *Journal of Speech and Hearing Research* 29, 75–81

Broen, P.A. (1972) The verbal environment of the language-learning child. *American Speech and Hearing Association Monographs* 17

Bronson, W. (1974) Mother-toddler interaction: a perspective on studying the development of competence. *Merrill-Palmer Quarterly of Behaviour and Development* 20, 275–301

Brown, A.L. and Murphy, M. (1975) Reconstruction of arbitrary logical sequences by preschool children. *Journal of Experimental Child Psychology* 20, 307–326

Brown, C.J. and Hurtig, R.R. (1983) Children's discourse competence: an evaluation of the development of inferential processes. *Discourse Processes* 6, 353–375

Brown, G. and Yule, G. (1983) *Discourse Analysis*. Cambridge: Cambridge University Press

Brown, R. (1973) *A First Language*. Cambridge, MA: Harvard University Press

Bruner, J.S. (1975) The ontogenesis of speech acts. *Journal of Child Language* 2, 1–19

Bruner, J.S. (1978) Berlyne Memorial Lecture. Acquiring the uses of language. *Canadian Journal of Psychology* 32, 204–218

Bruner, J.S. (1983) The acquisition of pragmatic commitments. In R.M. Golinkoff (ed.) *The Transition from Prelinguistic to Linguistic Communication*. Hillsdale, NJ: Lawrence Erlbaum

Bruner, J., Roy, C. and Ratner, N. (1982) The beginnings of request. In K.E. Nelson (ed.) *Children's Language*, Vol. 3. New York: Gardner Press

Bryan, T. (1974) An observational analysis of classroom behaviors of children with learning disabilities. *Journal of Learning Disabilities* 1, 23–34

Bryan, T. (1986) A review of studies on learning disabled children's communicative competence. In R.L. Schiefelbusch (ed.) *Language Competence: Assessment and Intervention*. Austin, Tx: Pro-Ed

Bryan, T. and Pflaum, S. (1978) Linguistic, cognitive and social analyses of learning disabled children's social interactions. *Learning Disability Quarterly* 1, 70–79

Bryan, T. and Wheeler, R. (1972) Perception of children with learning disabilities: the eye of the observer. *Journal of Learning Disabilities* 5, 484–488

Bryan, T., Donahue, M. and Pearl, R. (1981) Learning disabled children's peer interactions during a small group problem solving task. *Learning Disability Quarterly* 4, 13–22

Bryan, T., Donahue, M., Pearl, R. and Sturm, C. (1981) Learning disabled children's conversational skills: the T.V. Talk Show. *Learning Disability Quarterly* 1, 70–79

Buium, N., Rynders, J. and Turnure, J. (1973) Early maternal linguistic environment of normal and nonnormal language-learning children. *Proceedings of the 81st Annual Convention of the American Psychological Association*, 19–80

Bullowa, M. (ed.) (1979) *Before Speech: The Beginning of Interpersonal Communication*. Cambridge: Cambridge University Press

Camarata, S., Hughes, C. and Ruhl, K. (1988) Mild/moderate behaviorally disordered students: a population at risk for language disorders. *Language, Speech, and Hearing Services in Schools* 19, 191–200

Cantwell, D.P. and Baker, L. (1985) Interrelationship of communication, learning, and psychiatric disorders in children. In C. Simon (ed.) *Communication Skills and Classroom Success*, Vol. I: *Assessment*. San Diego, CA: College-Hill Press

Cardoso-Martins, C. and Mervis, C.B. (1985) Maternal speech to prelinguistic children with Down's syndrome. *American Journal of Mental Deficiency* 80, 451–158

Carter, A. (1978) From sensori-motor vocalizations to words: a case study of the evolution of attention-directing communication in the second year. In A. Lock (ed.) *Action, Gesture and Symbol: The Emergence of Language*. New York: Academic Press

Charniak, E. and McDermott, D. (1985) *Introduction to Artificial Intelligence*. Reading, MA: Addison-Wesley

Clark, E.V. and Andersen, E.S. (1979) Spontaneous repairs: awareness in the process of acquiring language. *Papers and Reports on Child Language Development*, No. 16, Stanford University

Cole, P. (1982) *Language Disorders in Preschool Children*. Englewood Cliffs, NJ: Prentice-Hall

Coleman, M. and Gilliberg, C. (1985) *The Biology of Autistic Syndromes*. New York: Praeger

Constable, C.M. (1983) Creating communicative context. In H. Winitz (ed.) *Treating Language Disorders*. Baltimore: University Park Press

Constable, C.M. (1986) The application of scripts in the organization of language intervention contexts. In K. Nelson (ed.) *Event Knowledge*. Hillsdale, NJ: Lawrence Erlbaum

Conti-Ramsden, G. (1990) Maternal recasts and other contingent replies to language-impaired children. *Journal of Speech and Hearing Disorders* 55, 262–274

Conti-Ramsden, G. and Friel-Patti, S. (1983) Mothers' discourse adjustments to language-impaired and non-language-impaired children. *Journal of Speech and Hearing Disorders* 48, 360–367

Conti-Ramsden, G. and Friel-Patti, S. (1984) Mother-child dialogues: a comparison of normal and language impaired children. *Journal of Communication Disorders* 17, 19–35

Conti-Ramsden, G. and Gunn, M. (1986) The development of conversational disability: a case study. *British Journal of Disorders of Communication* 21, 339–351

Corsaro, W.A. (1981) The development of social cognition in pre-school children: implications for language learning. *Topics in Language Disorders* **2**, 77–95

Cosgrove, J.M. and Patterson, C.J. (1977) Plans and the development of listener skills. *Developmental Psychology* **13**, 577–564

Coulthard, R.M. (1985) *An Introduction to Discourse Analysis*. London: Longman

Craig, H.K. (1983) Applications of pragmatic models for intervention. In T.M. Gallagher and C.A. Prutting (eds) *Pragmatic Assessment and Intervention Issues in Language*. San Diego, CA: College-Hill Press

Craig, H.K. and Evans, J.L. (1989) Turn exchange characteristics of SLI children's simultaneous and nonsimultaneous speech. *Journal of Speech and Hearing Disorders* **54**, 334–347

Cross, T. (1977) Mothers' speech adjustments: the contributions of selected child listener variables. In C.E. Snow and C.A. Ferguson (eds) *Talking to Children: Language Input and Acquisition*. Cambridge: Cambridge University Press

Cross, T. (1978) Mothers' speech and its association with rate of linguistic development in young children. In N. Waterson and C.E. Snow (eds) *The Development of Communication*. New York: Wiley

Cross, T. (1981) The linguistic experience of slow learners. In A.R.Nesdale, C. Pratt, R. Grieve, J. Field, D. Illingworth and J. Hogben (eds) *Advances in Child Development*. Proceedings of the First National Conference on Child Development, University of Western Australia, Nedlands

Cross, T. (1984) Habilitating the language-impaired child: ideas from studies of parent-child interaction. *Topics in Language Disorders* **4**, 1–14

Crystal, D. (1974) Review of R. Brown: *A First Language*. *Journal of Child Language* **1**, 287–307

Crystal, D. and Fletcher, P. (1979) Profile analysis of language disability. In C. Fillmore, D. Kempler and W.S-J. Wang (eds) *Individual Differences in Language Ability and Language Behaviour*. New York: Academic Press

Crystal, D., Fletcher, P. and Garman, M. (1976) *The Grammatical Analysis of Language Disability*, 2nd edn. San Diego: Singular Publishing Group

Cunningham, C.E., Reuler, E., Blackwell, J. and Deck, J. (1981) Behavioral and linguistic developments in the interactions of normal and retarded children with their mothers. *Child Development* **52**, 62–70

Demos, V. (1982) The role of affect in early childhood: an exploratory study. In E. Tronick (ed.) *Social Interchange in Infancy: Affect, Cognition, and Communication*. Baltimore, MD: University Park Press

Dewart, H. and Summers, S. (1988) *The Pragmatics Profile of Early Communication Skills*. London: NFER

Dickson, W.P. (1982) Two decades of referential communication research: a review and meta-analysis. In C.J. Brainerd and H. Pressley (eds) *Verbal Processes in Children: Progress in Cognitive Development Research*. New York: Springer Verlag

Donahue, M. (1981) Requesting strategies of learning disabled children. *Applied Psycholinguistics* **2**, 213–234

Donahue, M. (1987) Interactions between linguistic and pragmatic development in learning-disabled children: three views of the state of the union. In S. Rosenberg (ed.) *Advances in Applied Psycholinguistics*, Vol. 1: *Disorders of First Language Development*. Cambridge: Cambridge University Press

Donahue, M. and Bryan, T. (1983) Conversational skills and modeling in learning disabled boys. *Applied Psycholinguistics* **4**, 251-278

Donahue, M, Pearl, R. and Bryan, T. (1980) Learning disabled children's conversational competence: responses to inadequate messages. *Applied Psycholinguistics* **1**, 387–403

Donahue, M., Pearl, R. and Bryan, T. (1982) Learning disabled children's syntactic proficiency during a communicative task. *Journal of Speech and Hearing Disorders* **47**, 397–403

Donaldson, M. (1978) *Children's Minds*. London:Fontana

Donaldson, M. (1986) *Children's Explanations*. Cambridge: Cambridge University Press

Dore, J. (1983) Feeling, form, and intention in the baby's transition to language. In R.M. Golinkoff (ed.) *The Transition from Prelinguistic to Linguistic Communication*. Hillsdale, NJ: Lawrence Erlbaum

Duncan, S. (1972) Some signals and rules for taking speaking turns in conversation. *Journal of Personality and Social Psychology* **23**, 283–292

Durkin, K. (1987) Minds and language: social cognition, social interaction, and the acquisition of language. *Mind and Language* **2**, 105–140

Eheart, B.K. (1982) Mother–child interactions with non-retarded and mentally retarded preschoolers. *American Journal of Mental Deficiency* **87**, 20–25

Eisenberg, A.R. (1985) Learning to describe past experiences in conversation. *Discourse Processes* **8**, 177–204

Ellis, A. and Beattie, G. (1986) *The Psychology of Language and Communication*. London: Weidenfeld & Nicolson

Ervin-Tripp, S. (1977) Wait for me, roller-skate. In S.Ervin-Tripp and C.Mitchell-Kernan (eds) (1977) *Child Discourse*. New York: Academic Press

Ervin-Tripp, S. (1979) Children's verbal turn-taking. In E.Ochs and B.Schieffelin (eds) *Developmental Pragmatics*. New York: Academic Press

Ervin-Tripp, S. and Gordon, D. (1984) The development of requests. In R.L.Schiefelbusch (ed.) *Language Competence: Assessment and Intervention*. London: Taylor & Francis

Ervin-Tripp, S. and Mitchell-Kernan, C. (eds) (1977) *Child Discourse*. New York: Academic Press

Evans, M. (1985) Self-initiated speech repairs: a reflection of communication monitoring in young children. *Developmental Psychology* **21**, 365–371

Fay, W.H. and Schuler, A.L. (1980) *Emerging Language in Autistic Children*. London: Edward Arnold

Feagans, L. and Short, E. (1984) Developmental differences in the comprehension and production of narratives by reading disabled and normally achieving children. *Child Development* **55**, 1727–1736

Fein, G. (1981) Pretend play in childhood: an integrative review. *Child Development* **52**, 1095–1118

Fernald, A. (1984) The perceptual and affective salience of mothers' speech to infants. In L. Feagans, C. Garvey and R.M. Golinkoff (eds) *The Origins and Growth of Communication*. New York: Academic Press

Fey, M.E. (1986) *Language Intervention with Young Children*. San Diego, CA: College-Hill Press

Fey, M.E. and Leonard, L.B. (1983) Pragmatic skills of children with specific language impairment. In T.M. Gallagher and C.A. Prutting (eds) *Pragmatic Assessment and Intervention Issues in Language*. San Diego, CA: College-Hill Press

Fey, M.E., Leonard, L. and Wilcox, K. (1981) Speech style modification of language disordered children. *Journal of Speech and Hearing Disorders* **46**, 91–96

Fischer, M.A. (1983) An analysis of preverbal communicative behaviour in Down's syndrome and non-retarded children. Unpublished PhD thesis, University of Oregon

Fischer, M.A. (1987) Mother–child interaction in preverbal children with Down syndrome. *Journal of Speech and Hearing Disorders* **52**, 179–190

Flavell, J.H., Botkin, P.T., Fry, C.L.Jr., Wright, J.W. and Jarvis, P.E. (1968) *The Development of Role-taking and Communication Skills in Children*. New York: Wiley

Flavell, J.H., Speer, J.R., Green, F.L. and August, D.L. (1981) The development of comprehension monitoring and knowledge about communication. *Monographs of the Society for Research in Child Development* **46**, (5), 1–5

Fletcher, P. and Garman, M. (1988) Normal language development and language impairment: syntax and beyond. *Clinical Linguistics* **2**, 97–113

Foster, S. (1986) Learning discourse topic management in the preschool years. *Journal of Child Language* **13**, 231–250

Frith, U. (1989a) A new look at language and communication in autism. *British Journal of Disorders of Communication* **24**, 123–150

Frith, U. (1989b) *Autism: Explaining the Enigma*. Oxford: Basil Blackwell

Furrow, D. and Lewis, S. (1988) The role of the initial utterance in contingent query sequences: its influence on responses to requests for clarification. *Journal of Child Language* **14**, 467–479

Furrow, D., Nelson, K. and Benedict, H. (1979) Mothers' speech to children and syntactic development: some simple relationships. *Journal of Child Language* **6**, 423–442

Gallagher, T.M. (1977) Revision behaviors in the speech of normal children developing language. *Journal of Speech and Hearing Research* **20**, 303–318

Gallagher, T.M. (1981) Contingent query sequences within adult-child discourse. *Journal of Child Language* **8**, 51–62

Gallagher, T.M. (1983) Pre-assessment: a procedure for accommodating language use variability. In T.M. Gallagher and C.A. Prutting (eds) *Pragmatic Assessment and Intervention Issues in Language*. San Diego, CA: College-Hill Press

Gallagher, T.M. and Craig, H.K. (1982) An investigation of overlap in children's speech. *Journal of Psycholinguistic Research* **11**, 63–75

Gallagher, T.M. and Darnton, B. (1978) Conversational aspects of the speech of language disordered children: revision behaviors. *Journal of Speech and Hearing Research* **21**, 118–135

Gallagher, T.M. and Prutting, C.A. (eds) (1983) *Pragmatic Assessment and Intervention Issues in Language*. San Diego, CA: College-Hill Press

Garnham, A. (1985) *Psycholinguistics: Central Topics*. London: Methuen

Garnica, O.K. (1977) Some prosodic and paralinguistic features of speech to young children. In C.E. Snow and C.A. Ferguson (eds) *Talking to Children: Language Input and Acquisition*. Cambridge: Cambridge University Press

Garton, A.F. and Pratt, C. (1990) Children's pragmatic judgements of direct and indirect requests. *First Language* **10**, 51–59

Garvey, C. (1975) Requests and responses in children's speech. *Journal of Child Language* **2**, 41–63

Garvey, C. (1977) The contingent query: A dependent act in conversation. In M.Lewis and L.A.Rosenblum (eds) *Interaction, Conversation, and the Development of Language*. New York: Wiley

Garvey, C. and Berninger, G. (1981) Timing and turn-taking in children's conversations. *Discourse Processes* 4, 27–57

German, D. (1979) Word-finding skills in children with learning disabilities. *Journal of Learning Disabilities* 12, 176–181

Gleason, J.Berko (1975) Fathers and other strangers: men's speech to young children. In D.Dato (ed.) *Developmental Psycholinguistics: Theory and Application.* Washington, DC: Georgetown University Press

Gleason, J.Berko and Weintraub, S. (1976) The acquisition of routines in child language. *Language in Society* 5, 129–136

Gleitman, L.R., Newport, E.L. and Gleitman, H. (1984) The current status of the motherese hypothesis. *Journal of Child Language* 11, 43–79

Goldfield, B. (1985) The contribution of child and caregiver to individual differences in language acquisition. Unpublished doctoral dissertation: Harvard Graduate School of Education

Golinkoff, R.M. (ed.) (1983a) *The Transition from Prelinguistic to Linguistic Communication.* Hillsdale, NJ: Lawrence Erlbaum

Golinkoff, R.M. (ed.)(1983b) The preverbal negotiation of failed messages: insights into the transition period. In *The Transition from Prelinguistic to Linguistic Communication.* Hillsdale, NJ: Lawrence Erlbaum

Golinkoff, R.M. (1986) I beg your pardon? the preverbal negotiation of failed messages. *Journal of Child Language* 13, 455–476

Golinkoff, R.M. and Gordon, L. (1988) What makes communication run? Characteristics of immediate successes? *First Language* 8, 103–124

Gottman, J.M. and Parker, J.G. (1986) *Conversations of Friends: Speculations on Affective Development.* Cambridge: Cambridge University Press

Green, G.M. (1989) *Pragmatics and Natural Language Understanding.* Hillsdale, NJ: Lawrence Erlbaum

Greenfield, P.M. (1980) Toward an operational and logical analysis of intentionality: the use of discourse in early child language. In D. Olson (ed.) *The Social Foundations of Language and Thought.* New York: Norton

Greenlee, M. (1981) Learning to tell the forest from the trees: unravelling discourse features of a psychotic child. *First Language* 2, 83–102

Greenwald, C. and Leonard, L. (1979) Communicative and sensorimotor development of Down's syndrome children. *American Journal of Mental Deficiency* 84, 296–303

Grice, H.P. (1968) Utterer's meaning, sentence-meaning, and word-meaning. *Foundations of Language* 4, 1–18

Grice, H.P. (1975) Logic and conversation. In P. Cole and J.L. Morgan (eds) *Syntax and Semantics,* Vol. 3: *Speech Acts.* New York: Academic Press

Guralnick, M. and Paul-Brown, D. (1984) Communicative adjustments during behavior-request episodes among children at different developmental levels. *Child Development* 55, 911–919

Guralnick, M. and Paul-Brown, D. (1986) Communicative interactions of mildly delayed and normally developing preschool children: Effects of listener's developmental age. *Journal of Speech and Hearing Research* 29, 2–11

Gutfreund, M., Harrison, M. and Wells, G. (1989) *Bristol Language Development Scales.* Windsor, Berks: NFER-Nelson

Halliday, M.A.K. (1975) *Learning How to Mean.* London: Edward Arnold

Hansson, K. and Nettelbladt, U. (1990) The verbal interaction of Swedish language-disordered pre-school children. *Clinical Linguistics and Phonetics* 4, 39–48

Harding, C. (1983) Setting the stage for language acquisition: communication development in the first year. In R.M. Golinkoff (ed.) *The Transition from Prelinguistic to Linguistic Communication*. Hillsdale, NJ: Lawrence Erlbaum

Harding, C. and Golinkoff, R.M. (1979) The origins of intentional vocalizations in prelinguistic infants. *Child Development* 50, 33–40

Hargie, O., Saunders, C. and Dickson, D. (1987) *Social Skills and Interpersonal Communication*. London: Routledge

Hargrove, P.M., Straka, E.M. and Medders, E.G. (1988) Clarification requests of normal and language-impaired children. *British Journal of Disorders of Communication* 23, 51–62

Harris, M., Jones, D. and Grant, J. (1983) The nonverbal context of mothers' speech to infants. *First Language* 4, 21–30

Harris, M., Jones, D. and Grant, J. (1984) The social-interactional context of maternal speech to infants: an explanation for the event-bound nature of early word use. *First Language* 5, 89–100

Harris, M., Jones, D., Brookes, S. and Grant, J. (1986) Relations between the non-verbal context of maternal speech and rate of language development. *British Journal of Developmental Psychology* 4, 261–168

Haviland, S.E. and Clark, H.H. (1974) What's new? Acquiring new information as a process in comprehension. *Journal of Verbal Learning and Verbal Behavior* 13, 512–521

Hildyard, A. (1979) Children's production of inferences from oral texts. *Discourse Processes* 2, 33–56

Hirsch-Pasek, K. and Treiman, R. (1982) Doggerel: Motherese in a new context. *Journal of Child Language* 9, 229–237

Hobson, R.P. (1986a) The autistic child's appraisal of expressions of emotion. *Journal of Child Psychology and Psychiatry* 27, 321–342

Hobson, R.P. (1986b) The autistic child's appraisal of expressions of emotion: a further study. *Journal of Child Psychology and Psychiatry* 27, 671–680

Hobson, R.P., Ouston, J. and Lee, A. (1988a) What's in a face? The case of autism. *British Journal of Psychology* 79, 441–453

Hobson, R.P., Ouston, J. and Lee, A. (1988b) Emotion recognition in autism: co-ordinating faces and voices. *Psychological Medicine* 18, 911–923

Hoffman, M.L. (1981) Perspectives on the difference between understanding people and understanding things. In J.H. Flavell and L. Ross (eds) *Social Cognitive Development*. Cambridge: Cambridge University Press

Hopmann, M.R. and Maratsos, M.P. (1978) A developmental study of factivity and negation in complex syntax. *Journal of Child Language* 5, 295–309

Horsborough, K., Cross, T. and Ball, J. (1985) Conversational interaction between mothers and their autistic, dysphasic and normal children. In T.G. Cross and L.M. Riach (eds) *Issues and Research in Child Development*. Proceedings of the Second National Child Development Conference, The Institute of Early Childhood Development and Melbourne College of Advanced Education, Victoria, Australia

Howlin, P. (1980) The home treatment of autistic children. In L.A. Hersov, M. Berger and A.R. Nicol (eds) *Language and Language Disorders in Childhood*. New York: Pergamon Press

Humphreys, A. (1987) Recent research into autism: 1984–1986. *Communication* 21, 14–17

Hurtig, R., Ensrud, S. and Tomblin, J.B. (1982) The communicative function of question production in autistic children. *Journal of Autism and Developmental*

Disorders **12**, 57–69

Hutt, E. (1986) *Teaching Language-disordered Children: A Structured Curriculum.* London: Edward Arnold

Ironsmith, M. and Whitehurst, G.J. (1978) The development of listener abilities in communication: how children deal with ambiguous information. *Child Development* **49**, 348–352

Jackson, S. and Jacobs, S. (1982) Ambiguity and implicature in children's discourse comprehension. *Journal of Child Language* **9**, 209–216

Johnson, C.E. (1980) Contingent queries: the first chapter. In H. Giles, W. Robinson and P. Smith (eds) *Language: Social Psychological Perspectives.* Oxford: Pergamon

Johnston, J.R. (1985) The discourse symptoms of developmental disorders. In T. van Dijk (ed.) *Handbook of Discourse Analysis*, Vol. III. London: Academic Press

Jones, O.H.M. (1977) Mother-child communication sills in Down's syndrome and normal infants. In H.R. Schaffer (ed.) *Studies in Mother–Infant Interaction.* London: Academic Press

Jones, O.H.M. (1980) Prelinguistic communication skills in Down's syndrome and normal infants. In T. Field (ed.) *High-risk Infants and Children: Adult and Peer Interactions.* London: Academic Press

Kagan, J. (1984) *The Nature of the Child.* New York: Basic Books

Kamhi, A.G. and Johnston, J. (1982) Towards an understanding of retarded children's linguistic deficiencies. *Journal of Speech and Hearing Research* **25**, 435–445

Kamhi, A.G. and Masterson, J.J. (1989) Language and cognition in the mentally handicapped: last rites for the difference-delay controversy. In M. Beveridge, G. Conti-Ramsden and I.Leudar (eds) *Language and Communication in Mentally Handicapped Children.* London: Routledge, Chapman & Hall

Kanner, L. (1943) Autistic disturbances of affective contact. *Nervous Child* **2**, 217–250

Karmiloff-Smith, A. (1979) *A Functional Approach to Child Language.* Cambridge: Cambridge University Press

Kaye, K. (1977) Towards the origin of dialogue. In H.R. Schaffer (ed.) *Studies in Mother–Child Interaction.* New York: Academic Press

King, M.F. (1989) Development of pragmatic skills in children with moderate learning difficulty. MSc Dissertation in General and Applied Linguistics, University of Ulster at Jordanstown

Kiparsky, P. and Kiparsky, C. (1970) Fact. In D. Steinberg and L. Jakobovits (eds) *Semantics: An Interdisciplinary Reader.* Cambridge: Cambridge University Press

Klee, T. and Fitzgerald, M.D. (1985) The relation between grammatical development and mean length of utterance in morphemes. *Journal of Child Language* **12**, 251–269

Klee, T., Schaffer, M., May, S., Membrino, I. and Mougey, K. (1989) A comparison of the age-MLU relation in normal and specifically language-impaired preschool children. *Journal of Speech and Hearing Disorders* **54**, 226–233

Krauss, R.M. and Glucksberg, S. (1969) The development of communication: competence as a function of age. *Child Development* **40**, 255–266

Kysela, G.M., Holdgrafer, G., McCarthy, C. and Stewart, T. (1990) Turntaking and pragmatic language skills of developmentally delayed children: a research note. *Journal of Communication Disorders* **23**, 135–149

Labov, W. and Fanshel, D. (1977) *Therapeutic Discourse: Psychotherapy as Conversation.* New York: Academic Press

Landry, S. H. and Loveland, K.A. (1988) Communication behaviors in autism and developmental language delay. *Journal of Child Psychology and Psychiatry* **29**, 621–634

Lasky, E.Z. and Klopp, K. (1982) Parent-child interactions in normal and language-disordered children. *Journal of Speech and Hearing Disorders* **47**, 7–18

Launer, P.B. and Lahey, M. (1981) Passages: from the fifties to the eighties in language assessment. *Topics in Language Disorders* **1**, 11–29

Ledbetter, P.J. and Dent, C.H. (1988) Young children's sensitivity to direct and indirect request structure. *First Language* **8**, 227–246

Leech, G. (1983) *Pragmatics.* London: Longman

Leifer, J.S. and Lewis, M. (1984) Acquisition of conversational response skills by young Down syndrome and non-retarded young children. *American Journal of Mental Deficiency* **88**, 610–618

Leonard, L.B. (1981) Facilitating linguistic skills in children with specific language impairment. *Applied Psycholinguistics* **2**, 89–118

Leonard, L. (1983) Speech selection and modification in language-disordered children. *Topics in Language Disorders* **4** (1), 28–37

Leonard, L. (1986) Conversational replies of children with specific language impairment. *Journal of Speech and Hearing Research* **29**, 114–119

Leonard, L., Camarata, S., Rowan, L. and Chapman, K. (1982) The communicative functions of lexical usage by language-impaired children. *Applied Psycholinguistics* **3**, 109–127

Leslie, A.M. (1987) Pretence and representation: the origins of 'theory of mind'. *Psychological Review* **94**, 412–426

Letts, C. (1985) Linguistic interaction in the clinic: how do therapists do therapy? *Child Language Teaching and Therapy* **3**, 321–331

Letts, C. (1989) Exploring therapy and classroom interaction. In P. Grunwell and A. James (eds) *The Functional Evaluation of Language Disorders.* London: Croom Helm

Leudar, I. (1981) Strategic communication in mental retardation. In W.I. Frazer and R.Grieve (eds) *Communication with Normal and Retarded Children.* Bristol: Wright

Levin, E.A. and Rubin, K.H. (1983) Getting others to do what you want them to do: the development of children's requestive strategies. In K.E. Nelson (ed.) *Children's Language,* Vol. 4. Hillsdale, NJ: Lawrence Erlbaum

LeVine, R. (1977) Child rearing as cultural adaptation. In P.H. Liederman, S. Tulkin and A. Rosenfeld (eds) *Culture and Infancy: Variations in the Human Experience.* Orlando, Florida: Academic Press

Levinson, S. (1983) *Pragmatics.* Cambridge: Cambridge University Press

Light, P. (1979) *The Development of Social Sensitivity.* Cambridge: Cambridge University Press

Liles, B. (1985a) Cohesion in the narratives of normal and language-disordered children. *Journal of Speech and Hearing Research* **28**, 123–133

Liles, B. (1985b) Production and comprehension of narrative discourse in normal and language-disordered children. *Journal of Communication Disorders* **18**, 409–427

Lloyd, P. and Beveridge, M. (1981) *Information and Meaning in Child Communication.* New York: Academic Press

Lock, A. (ed.)(1978) *Action, Gesture and Symbol: The Emergence of Language.* New York: Academic Press

Longhurst, T.M. (1974) Communication in retarded adolescents: sex and intelligence level. *American Journal of Mental Deficiency* **78**, 607–618

Longhurst, T. and Stepanich, L. (1975) Mothers' speech addressed to one-, two-, and three-year-old normal children. *Child Study Journal* **5**, 3–11

McCaleb, P. and Prizant, B.M. (1985) Encoding of new versus old information by autistic children. *Journal of Speech and Hearing Disorders* 50, 230–240

MacLachlan, B.G. and Chapman, R.S. (1988) Communication breakdowns in normal and language learning-disabled children's conversation and narration. *Journal of Speech and Hearing Disorders* 53, 2–7

McLaughlin, M.L. (1984) *Conversation: How Talk is Organised*. Beverly Hills: Sage

MacPherson, C.A. and Weber-Olsen, M. (1980) Mother speech input to deficient and language normal children. *Proceedings from the First Wisconsin Symposium on Research on Child Language Disorders* 1, 59–79

McTear, M. (1985a) *Children's Conversation*. Oxford: Blackwell

McTear, M. (1985b) Pragmatic disorders: a case study of conversational disability. *British Journal of Disorders of Communication* 20, 129–141

McTear, M. (1987) *The Articulate Computer*. Oxford: Blackwell

McTear, M. (1989) Semantic-pragmatic disability: a disorder of thought? In D.M.Topping, D.C. Crowell and V.N. Kobayashi (eds) *Thinking Across Cultures: The Third International Conference on Thinking*. Hillsdale, NJ: Lawrence Erlbaum

Mann, J. and Mann, C. (1966) The effect of role-playing experience on role-playing ability. In B. Biddle and E. Thomas (eds) *Role Theory: Concepts and Research*. New York: Wiley & Sons

Maratsos, M.P. (1973) Nonegocentric communication abilities in preschool children. *Child Development* 44, 697–700

Maratsos, M.P. and Chalkley, M. (1981) The internal language of children's syntax: the ontogenesis and representation of syntactic categories. In K.E.Nelson (ed.) *Children's Language, Vol. 2*. New York: Gardner Press

Markman, E. (1977) Realizing that you don't understand: a preliminary investigation. *Child Development* 48, 986–992

Markman, E. (1981) Comprehension monitoring. In W.P.Dickson (ed.) *Children's Oral Communication Skills*. New York: Academic Press

Marshall, N.R., Hegrenes, J.R. and Goldstein, S. (1973) Verbal interactions: mothers and their retarded children vs. mothers and their non-retarded children. *American Journal of Mental Deficiency* 77, 415–419

Meline, T.J. (1986) Referential communication skills of learning disabled/language impaired children. *Applied Psycholinguistics* 7, 129–140

Meline, T.J. (1988) The encoding of novel referents by language-impaired children. *Language, Speech and Hearing Services in Schools* 19, 119–127

Milford, S.A. (1989) Children's acquisition of the presuppositional status of factive and non-factive verbs. MSc Dissertation in General and Applied Linguistics, University of Ulster at Jordanstown

Miller, C.L. and Byrne, J.M. (1984) The role of temporal cues in the development of language and communication. In L. Feagans, C. Garvey and R.M. Golinkoff (eds) *The Origins and Growth of Communication*. New York: Academic Press

Miller, J.F. (1981) *Assessing Language Production in Children*. Baltimore: University Park Press

Minsky, M.(ed.)(1968) Matter, mind and models. In *Semantic Information Processing*. Cambridge, MA: MIT Press

Mirenda, P.L., Donnellan, A. and Yoder, D.E. (1983) Gaze behavior: a new look at an old problem. *Journal of Autism and Developmental Disorders* 13, 397–409

Mitchell-Kernan, C. and Kernan, K.T. (1977) Functional considerations in the choice of directive forms by black American children. In S.Ervin-Tripp and C.Mitchell-Kernan (eds) *Child Discourse*. New York: Academic Press

Morehead, D. and Ingram, D. (1976) The development of base syntax in normal and linguistically deviant children. In D. Morehead and A. Morehead (eds) *Normal and Deficient Child Language*. Baltimore: University Park Press

Muma, J. (1978) *Language Handbook: Concepts, Assessment, Intervention*. Englewood Cliffs, NJ: Prentice-Hall

Muma, J.R. (1983) Speech-language pathology: emerging clinical expertise in language. In T. Gallagher and C. Prutting (eds) *Pragmatic Assessment and Intervention Issues in Language*. San Diego, CA: College-Hill Press

Nelson, K. (1973) *Structure and Strategy in Learning How to Talk*. Monographs of the Society for Research in Child Development, No. 149, Vol. 38

Nelson, K.(1986) *Event Knowledge*. Hillsdale, NJ: Lawrence Erlbaum

Nelson, K. and Gruendel, J.M. (1979) At morning it's lunchtime: a scriptal view of children's dialogues. *Discourse Processes* 2, 73–94

Nelson, K.E. (1977) Facilitating children's syntax acquisition. *Developmental Psychology* 13, 101–107

Nelson, K.E. (1981) Toward a rare-event cognitive comparison theory of syntax acquisition: insights from work with recasts. In P. Dale and D. Ingram (eds) *Child Language: An International Perspective*. Baltimore: University Park Press

Nelson, K.E., Bonvillian, J., Denninger, M., Kaplan, B. and Baker, N. (1984) Maternal input adjustments and nonadjustments as related to children's linguistic advances and to language acquisition theories. In A. Pellegrini and T. Yawkey (eds) *The Development of Oral and Written Language in Social Contexts*. Norwood, NJ: Ablex

Newhoff, M. and Browning, J. (1983) Interactional variation: a view from the language-disordered child's world. *Topics in Language Disorders* 4, 49–60

Newhoff, M., Silverman, L. and Millet, A. (1980) Linguistic differences in parents' speech to normal and language disordered children. *Proceedings from the First Wisconsin Symposium on Research in Child Language Disorders* 1, 44–57

Newport, E.L., Gleitman, L.R. and Gleitman, H. (1977) Mother, I'd rather do it myself: some effects and noneffects of maternal speech style. In C.E. Snow and C.A. Ferguson (eds) *Talking to Children: Language Input and Acquisition*. Cambridge: Cambridge University Press

Noel, N.M. (1980) Referential communication abilities of learning disabled children. *Learning Disability Quarterly* 3, 70–75

Norris, J.A. and Damico, J.S. (1990) Whole language in theory and practice: implications for language intervention. *Language, Speech, and Hearing Services in Schools* 21, 212–220

Ochs, E. (1979) Introduction: what child language can contribute to pragmatics. In E.Ochs and B.Schieffelin (eds) *Developmental Pragmatics*. New York: Academic Press

Ochs, E. and Schieffelin, B. (eds) (1979) *Developmental Pragmatics*. New York: Academic Press

Ochs, E. and Schieffelin, B.B. (1984) Language acquisition and socialization: three developmental stories and their implications. In R. Schweder and R. LeVine (eds) *Cultural Theory: Essays on Mind, Self and Emotion*. Cambridge: Cambridge University Press

Oden, S. and Asher, S. (1977) Coaching children in social skills for friendship making. *Child Development* 48, 495–506

Olson, D.R. (1970) Language acquisition and cognitive development. In H.C.Haywood (ed.) *Social–Cultural Aspects of Mental Retardation*. New York: Appleton–Century–Crofts

Olson, D.R. and Nickerson, N.G. (1979) Language development through the school years. In K.E. Nelson (ed.) *Children's Language*, Vol. 1. New York: Gardner Press

Owen, R.E. and MacDonald, J.D. (1982) Communicative uses of the early speech of nondelayed and Down syndrome children. *American Journal of Mental Deficiency* 86, 503–510

Paccia, J.M. and Curcio, F. (1982) Language processing and forms of immediate echolalia in autistic children. *Journal of Speech and Hearing Research* 25, 42–47

Pace, A.J. and Feagans, L. (1984) Knowledge and language: children's ability to use and communicate what they know about everyday experiences. In L.Feagans, C. Garvey and R.M. Golinkoff (eds) *The Origins and Growth of Communication*. New York: Academic Press

Paris, S.G. and Mahoney, G.J. (1974) Cognitive integration in children's memory for sentences and pictures. *Child Development* 45, 633–642

Pearl, R., Donahue, M. and Bryan, T. (1983) Learning disabled and normal children's responses to non–explicit requests for clarification. *Perceptual and Motor Skills* 53, 919–925

Pearl, R., Donahue, M. and Bryan, T. (1985) The development of tact: children's strategies for delivering bad news. *Journal of Applied Developmental Psychology* 6, 141–149

Perner, J. (1988) Higher-order beliefs and intentions in children's understanding of social interaction. In J.W. Astington, P.L. Harris and D.R. Olson (eds) *Developing Theories of Mind*. Cambridge: Cambridge University Press

Perner, J. and Wimmer, H. (1985) "John thinks that Mary thinks that..." Attribution of second-order beliefs by 5- to 10-year-old children. *Journal of Experimental Child Psychology* 39, 437–471

Petersen, G.A. and Sherrod, K.B. (1982) Relationship of maternal language to language development and language delay in children. *American Journal of Mental Deficiency* 86, 391–398

Phillips, J. (1973) Syntax and vocabulary of mothers' speech to young children: Age and sex comparisons. *Child Development* 44, 182–185

Piaget, J. (1926) *The Language and Thought of the Child*. London: Routledge

Porter, R. and Conti-Ramsden, G. (1987) Clarification requests and the language-impaired child. *Child Language Teaching and Therapy* 3, 133–150

Prinz, P.M. (1982) An investigation of the comprehension and production of requests in normal and language-disordered children. *Journal of Communication Disorders* 15, 75–93

Prinz, P.M. and Ferrier, L. (1983) "Can you give me that one?": the comprehension, production and judgement of directives in language-impaired children. *Journal of Speech and Hearing Disorders* 48, 44–54

Prior, H., Minnes, P., Coyne, T., Golding, B., Hendy, J. and McGillivray, J. (1979) Verbal interactions between staff and residents in an institution for the young mentally retarded. *Mental Retardation* 17, 65–70

Prizant, B.M., Audet, L.R., Burke, G.M., Hummel, L.J. and Maher, S.R. (1990) Communication disorders and emotional/behavioral disorders in children and adolescents. *Journal of Speech and Hearing Disorders* 55, 179–192

Prutting, C.A. (1982) Pragmatics as social competence. *Journal of Speech and Hearing Disorders* 47, 123–134

Prutting, C.A. and Kirchner, D.M. (1983) Applied pragmatics. In T.M. Gallagher and

C.A. Prutting (eds) *Pragmatic Assessment and Intervention Issues in Language*. San Diego, CA: College-Hill Press

Prutting, C.A. and Kirchner, D.M. (1987) A clinical appraisal of the pragmatic aspects of language. *Journal of Speech and Hearing Disorders* **52**, 105–119

Prutting, C.A., Bagshaw, N., Goldstein, H., Juskowitz, S. and Umen, E. (1978) Clinician-child discourse: some preliminary questions. *Journal of Speech and Hearing Disorders* **43**, 123–139

Ramey, C.T., Sparling, J.J. and Wasik, B.H. (1981) Creating social environments to facilitate language development. In R. Schiefelbusch and D. Bricker (eds) *Early Language: Acquisition and Intervention*. Baltimore: University Park Press

Rapin, I. and Allen, D.A. (1983) Developmental language disorders: Nosologic considerations. In U.Kirk (ed.) *Neuropsychology of Language, Reading and Spelling*. New York: Academic Press

Rapin, I. and Allen, D.A. (1986) Communication disorders of early childhood: attempts at classification. In I. Flehmig and L. Stern (eds) *Child Development and Learning Behavior*. New York: Gustav Fisher Verlag

Rapin, I. and Allen, D.A. (1987) Developmental dysphasia and autism in preschool children: characteristics and subtypes. *Proceedings of the First International Symposium on Specific Speech and Language Disorders in Children*, pp. 20–35. Available from: Association for all Speech Impaired Children (AFASIC)

Read, B.K. and Cherry, L.J. (1978) Preschool children's production of directive forms. *Discourse Processes* **1**, 233–245

Reeder, K. (1980) The emergence of illocutionary skills. *Journal of Child Language* **7**, 13–28

Richards, M.P.M. (ed.)(1974) First steps in becoming social. In *The Integration of a Child into a Social World*. Cambridge: Cambridge University Press

Ricks, D.M. (1975) Vocal communication in pre-verbal normal and autistic children. In N. O'Connor (ed.) *Language, Cognitive Deficits and Retardation*. London: Butterworths

Ricks, D.M. and Wing, L. (1975) Language, communication, and the use of symbols in normal and autistic children. *Journal of Autism and Childhood Schizophrenia* **5**, 191–221

Ripich, D.N. and Spinelli, F.M. (1985) An ethnographic approach to assessment and intervention. In D.N. Ripich and F.M. Spinelli (eds) *School Discourse Problems*. San Diego: Singular Publishing Group

Robinson, E.J. (1981) The child's understanding of inadequate messages and communication failure: a problem of ignorance or egocentrism? In W.P. Dickson (ed.) *Children's Oral Communication Skills*. New York: Academic Press

Robinson, E.J. and Robinson, W.P. (1977) Development in the understanding of causes of success and failure in verbal communication. *Cognition* **5**, 363–378

Rom, A. and Bliss, L.S. (1981) A comparison of verbal communicative skills of language impaired and normal speaking children. *Journal of Communication Disorders* **14**, 133–140

Rondal, J.A. (1977) Maternal speech to normal and Down's syndrome children matched for mean length of utterance. In E. Meyers (ed.) *Quality of Life in Severely and Profoundly Mentally Retarded People: Research Foundations for Improvement*. Washington DC: American Association of Mental Deficiency

Rosinski-McClendon, M.K. and Newhoff, M. (1987) Conversational responsiveness and assertiveness in language-impaired children. *Language, Speech and Hearing Services in Schools* **18**, 53–62

Roth, P.L. (1987) Temporal characteristics of maternal verbal styles. In K.E.Nelson and A.van Kleeck (eds) *Children's Language*, Vol. 6. Hillsdale, NJ: Lawrence Erlbaum

Roth, F.P. and Spekman, NJ (1984) Assessing the pragmatic ability of children: Part 1. Organisational framework and assessment parameters. *Journal of Speech and Hearing Disorders* 49, 2–11

Rubin, K. (1980) *Children's Play*. San Francisco, CA: Jossey-Bass

Rueda, R. and Chan, K.S. (1980) Referential communication skills levels of moderately mentally retarded adolescents. *American Journal of Mental Deficiency* 85, 45–52

Rumsey, J.M. and Hamburger, S.D. (1988) Neuropsychological findings in high functioning men with infantile autism, residual state. *Journal of Clinical and Experimental Neuropsychology* 10, 201–221

Rustin, L. and Kuhr, A. (1989) *Social Skills and the Speech Impaired*. London: Taylor & Francis.(Distributed in North America by Singular Publishing Group, San Diego, CA)

Rutter, M. (1978) Language disorder and infantile autism. In M. Rutter and E. Schopler (eds) *Autism: A Reappraisal of Concepts and Treatment*. New York: Plenum Press

Ryan, J. (1975) Mental subnormality and language development. In E.H.Lenneberg and E.Lenneberg (eds) *Foundations of Language Development*, Vol. II. London: Academic Press

Sachs, J. and Devin, J. (1976) Young children's use of age-appropriate speech styles in social interaction and role-playing. *Journal of Child Language* 3, 81–98

Sacks, H., Schegloff, E.A. and Jefferson, G. (1974) A simplest systematics for the organisation of turn-taking for conversation. *Language* 50, 696–735

Schaffer, H.R. (ed.) (1977) *Studies in Mother–Child Interaction*. New York: Academic Press

Schank, R.C. and Abelson, R.F. (1977) *Scripts, Plans, Goals, and Understanding*. Hillsdale, NJ: Lawrence Erlbaum

Schegloff, E.A. (1978) On some questions and ambiguities in conversation. In W.U. Dressler (ed.) *Current Trends in Textlinguistics*. Berlin: Walter de Gruyter

Schegloff, E.A. and Sacks, H. (1973) Opening up closings. *Semiotica* 8, 289–327

Schieffelin, B.B. (1984) *How Kaluli Children Learn What to Say, What to Do, and How to Feel: An Ethnographic Study of the Development of Communicative Competence*. Orlando, Florida: Academic Press

Scollon, R. (1976) *Conversations with a One Year Old*. Honolulu: University of Hawaii Press

Scoville, R.P. and Gordon, A.M. (1980) Children's understanding of factive presuppositions: an experiment and a review. *Journal of Child Language* 7, 381–399

Searle, J.R. (1969) *Speech Acts: An Essay in the Philosophy of Language*. Cambridge: Cambridge University Press

Shantz, C.U. (1981) The role of role-taking in children's referential communication. In W.P. Dickson (ed.) *Children's Oral Communication Skills*. New York: Academic Press

Shantz, C.U. (1983) Social cognition. In J.H. Flavell and E.M. Markman (eds) *Carmichael's Manual of Child Psychology*, Vol. 3, *Cognitive Development*. New York: Wiley

Shatz, M. (1978) Children's comprehension of their mothers' question-directives. *Journal of Child Language* 5, 39–46

Shatz, M. (1983a) On transition, continuity, and coupling: an alternative approach to communicative development. In R.M.Golinkoff (ed.) *The Transition from Prelinguistic to Linguistic Communication*. Hillsdale, NJ: Lawrence Erlbaum

Shatz, M. (1983b) Communication. In P.H.Mussen (ed.) *Handbook of Child Psychology*, 4th edn: Vol. 3: *Cognitive Development*. New York: Wiley

Shatz, M. and Gelman, R. (1973) The development of communication skills: modifications in the speech of young children as a function of listener. *Monographs of the Society for Research in Child Development* **38**, 5

Shatz, M., Bernstein, D. and Shulman, M. (1980) The responses of language disordered children to indirect directives in varying contexts. *Applied Psycholinguistics* **1**, 295–306

Shulman, B. (1985) *Test of Pragmatic Skills*. AZ: Communication Skill Builders

Silliman, E. (1984) Interactional competencies in the instructional context: the role of teaching discourse in learning. In G. Wallach and K. Butler (eds) *Language Learning Disabilities in School-age Children*. Baltimore, MD: Williams & Wilkins

Sinclair, J.M. and Coulthard, R.M. (1975) *Towards an Analysis of Discourse: The English used by Teachers and Pupils*. Oxford: Oxford University Press

Smedley, M. (1989) Semantic-pragmatic language disorder: a description with some practical suggestions for teachers. *Child Language Teaching and Therapy* **5**, 174–190

Smith, B.R. and Leinonen, E. (1991) *Clinical Pragmatics*. London: Chapman & Hall

Snow, C.E. (1972) Mothers' speech to children learning language. *Child Development* **43**, 549–565

Snow, C.E. (1977) The development of conversation between mothers and babies. *Journal of Child Language* **4**, 1–22

Snow, C.E. (1982) Are parents language teachers? In K. Borman (ed.) *The Social Life of Children in a Changing Society*. Hillsdale, NJ: Lawrence Erlbaum

Snow, C.E. and Ferguson, C.A. (eds) (1977) *Talking to Children: Language Input and Acquisition*. Cambridge: Cambridge University Press

Snow, C.E. and Goldfield, B.A. (1983) Turn the page please: Situation-specific language acquisition. *Journal of Child Language* **10**, 551–569

Snow, C.E., Perlmann, R. and Nathan, D. (1987) Why routines are different: Toward a multiple-factors model of the relation between input and language acquisition. In K.E. Nelson and A. van Kleeck (eds) *Children's Language*, Vol. 6. Hillsdale, NJ: Lawrence Erlbaum

Snow, C.E., Arlman-Rupp, A., Hassing, Y., Jobse, J., Joosten, J. and Vorster, J. (1976) Mothers' speech in three social classes. *Journal of Psycholinguistic Research* **5**, 1–20

Snow, C.E., Midkiff-Borunda, S., Small, A. and Proctor, A. (1984) Therapy as social interaction: Analyzing the contexts for language remediation. *Topics in Language Disorders* **4**, 72–85

Sonnenschein, S. and Whitehurst, G.J. (1980) The development of communication: when a bad model makes a good teacher. *Journal of Experimental Child Psychology* **29**, 371–390

Spekman, N. (1981) A study of the dyadic verbal communication abilities of learning disabled and normally achieving fourth and fifth grade boys. *Learning Disability Quarterly* **4**, 139–151

Spinelli, F.M. and Ripich, D.N. (eds)(1985) A comparison of classroom and clinical discourse. In *School Discourse Problems*. San Diego: Singular Publishing Group

Stella-Prorok, E.M. (1983) Mother–child language in the natural environment. In K.E.Nelson (ed.) *Children's Language*, Vol. 4. New York: Gardner Press

Stoneman, Z., Brody, G.H. and Abbott, D. (1983) In-home observations of young Down Syndrome children with their mothers and fathers. *American Journal of*

Mental Deficiency **87**, 591–600

Stubbs, M. (1983) *Discourse Analysis*. Oxford: Blackwell

Stubbs, M. (1986) *Educational Linguistics*. Oxford: Blackwell

Tager-Flusberg, H. (1981) On the nature of linguistic functioning in early infantile autism. *Journal of Autism and Developmental Disorders* **11**, 45–56

Terdal, L.E., Jackson, H.R. and Garner, A.M. (1975) Mother–child interactions: A comparison between normal and developmentally delayed groups. In E. Mash, L.A. Hammerlynck and L.C. Handy (eds) *Behaviour Modification and Families*. New York: Brunner/Mazel

Tomasello, M., Conti-Ramsden, G. and Ewert, B. (1990) Young children's conversations with their mothers and fathers: differences in breakdown and repair. *Journal of Child Language* **17**, 115–130

Trevarthen, C. (1979) Communication and co-operation in early infancy: a description of primary subjectivity. In M. Bullowa (ed.) *Before Speech: The Beginning of Interpersonal Communication*. Cambridge: Cambridge University Press

Trevarthen, C. and Hubley, P. (1978) Secondary subjectivity: confidence, confiding and acts of meaning in the first year. In A. Lock (ed.) *Action, Gesture and Symbol: The Emergence of Language*. New York: Academic Press

Van Kleeck, A. and Frankel, T. (1981) Discourse devices used by language disordered children. *Journal of Speech and Hearing Disorders* **46**, 250–257

Waterson, N. and Snow, C.E. (eds) (1978) *The Development of Communication*. New York: Wiley

Watson, M. (1981) The development of social roles: A sequence of social-cognitive development. *New Directions for Child Development* **12**, 33–41

Weintraub, S. and Mesulam, M.M. (1982) Developmental learning disabilities of the right hemisphere. *Archives of Neurology* **40**, 463–468

Wellman, H.M. and Lempers, J.D. (1977) The naturalistic communicative abilities of two-year-olds. *Child Development* **48**, 1052–1057

Wells, G. (1981) *Language through Interaction*. Cambridge: Cambridge University Press

Wetherby, A.M., Yonclas, D.C. and Bryan, A.A. (1989) Communicative profiles of preschool children with handicaps: implications for early identification. *Journal of Speech and Hearing Disorders* **54**, 148–158

Whitehurst, G.J. and Sonnenschein, S. (1981) The development of informative messages in referential communication: knowing when versus knowing how. In W.P.Dickson (ed.) *Children's Oral Communication Skills*. New York: Academic Press

Whitehurst, G.J., Sonnenschein, S. and Ianfolla, B.J. (1981) Learning to communicate from models: children confuse length with information. *Child Development* **52**, 507–513

Whiten, A. (1977) Assessing the effects of perinatal events on the success of the mother-infant relationship. In H.R.Schaffer (ed.) *Studies in Mother–Child Interaction*. New York: Academic Press

Wiig, E. and Semel, E. (1984) *Language Assessment and Intervention for the Learning Disabled*. Columbus: Merrill

Wimmer, H. and Perner, J. (1983) Beliefs about beliefs: representation and constraining function of wrong beliefs in young children's understanding of deception. *Cognition* **13**, 103-128

Wing, L (1981a) Language, social and cognitive impairments in autism and severe mental retardation. *Journal of Autism and Developmental Disorders* **11**, 31–44

Wing, L. (1981b) Asperger's syndrome: A clinical account. *Psychological Medicine* **11**, 115–129

Wing, L (1988) The continuum of autistic characteristics. In F. Shopler and G.B. Mesibov (eds) *Diagnosis and Assessment in Autism*. New York: Plenum Press

Wing, L. and Attwood, A. (1987) Syndromes of autism and atypical development. In D.J. Cohen, A. Donellan and R. Paul (eds) *Handbook of Autism and Pervasive Developmental Disorders*. New York: Wiley

Wing, L. and Gould, J. (1979) Severe impairments of social interaction and associated abnormalities in children: Epidemiology and classification. *Journal of Autism and Developmental Disorders* **9**, 11–29

Winitz, H. (1983) *Treating Language Disorders: For Clinicians by Clinicians*. Baltimore: University Park Press

Wulbert, M. Inglis, S., Kriegsmann, E. and Mills, B. (1975) Language delay and associated mother–child interaction. *Developmental Psychology* **11**, 61–70

Zahn-Waxler, C., Radke-Yarrow, M. and King, R. (1979) Child rearing and children's prosocial initiations towards victims of distress. *Child Development* **50**, 319–330